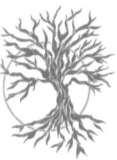

Why Are People Turning Green

Why Are People Turning Green

Seven Stories of Illness and Recovery;

The Impact of Toxins and Chemicals on the Mind and Body

Revised June 5 2017

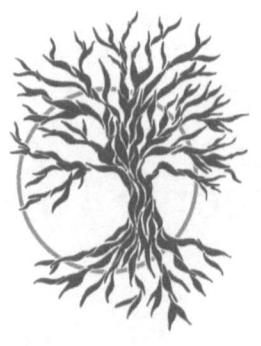

Cait Murphy MS LCMHC

Illustration & Cover - Erik Warn
Published by Eden Living PLLC

ISBN-13: 978-1542465137
ISBN-10: 1542465133

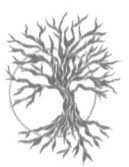

DEDICATION

In God I move and breathe and have my being.

This book is dedicated to:

My friend, partner, and love of my life: Without your love, support, encouragement and personal journey with this issue, the research project and book would not have been possible.

My sons: Jason, Erik and Patrick. I wish I knew this information when I was raising you. I would have made such different and healthier choices! To my grandchildren, Logan and Harper, in hopes of a healthier world for you.

The seven individuals who shared their story in the original research project: I truly appreciate your courage and dedication to this vitally important issue, and trust that your stories will encourage others to a path of health, wellness and recovery.

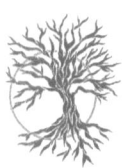

TABLE OF CONTENTS

INTRODUCTION

There is a common misconception that products sold to us are safe, and there is a pill for everything that ails us. It is my hope, after reading the stories of the seven people in this book, you will begin to consider that perhaps it is not the pill we add but the toxin we eliminate which will result in a better sense of health and wellbeing. The seven people presented in this book describe symptoms which commonly bring people to seek treatment in medical offices and mental health practices across the country. After months of frustration, unsuccessful results, and financial expense, these people took control of their lives and opted to heal themselves by avoiding culturally prominent chemicals and toxins.

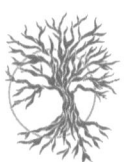

CHAPTER 1
IT'S PERSONAL

As a mental health counselor, I hear numerous stories every day from people struggling with emotional problems, chronic illness and/or chronic pain as well. They also report spending money and time they don't have, going from one appointment to another while experiencing little to no improvement. In some cases, the medications that have been prescribed to them have made matters worse creating negative side effects, exacerbated symptoms or addictions. People tell me they feel hopeless, angry, and helpless. They often feel blamed that somehow, it's their fault that they are sick, that it's all in their head, or that they're just "med seeking". This, of course, leaves them feeling that the system has failed them.

I was one of those people.

Before implementing major changes in my lifestyle habits, I had several health issues, some of which had followed me since childhood.   As a toddler, I suffered with respiratory illnesses.   I was hospitalized with pneumonia before I was 5 years old, and spent more than my share of time during the winter months, home sick in bed, while my friends were at school. I also had severe allergies, from dust, pollen, animals, trees, (life in general) which resulted in years of allergy shots, and being quarantined inside during the spring and fall, surrounded by boxes of tissues in an anti-histamine induced stupor.

As I entered high school, frequent headaches, dizziness, fainting spells, and digestive problems began. I am sure that diet pills, laxatives and use of antacids may have contributed to my problem.   I was convinced, by family history and the medical profession, that my gall bladder was the culprit. Tests always proved negative. Later in my adult life a "flare-up" sent me to the emergency room. After several tests and treatment options, I serendipitously ran into a nutritionist who told my symptoms sounded like a food intolerance. She suggested that I have a food sensitivity (not allergy) test.   A finger prick and several weeks later I discovered I had a severe insensitivity to eggs! Neither, I nor anyone else throughout my life, had ever considered this possibility. I had allergy testing as a child, and was allergic to a myriad of things, yet eggs, never showed up in any of those tests. After months of eliminating eggs from my diet, my

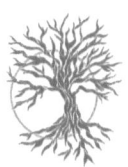

digestive issues significantly improved! I say, *significantly improved and not eliminated*, because I cheat now and again. When I am in strict adherence to the egg free regime, I have NO issues.

Along with allergies and digestive issues, I was often anxious and moody. During the summer of my 8th grade, I began experiencing long bouts of insomnia. Later as an adult, my mood swung from pleasant to irritable, to stressed and depressed back to elated. Yes, I was a joy to live with I'm sure. I do know that it felt horrible inside to be me; despite the medications I had been prescribed. Suddenly, for no reason, I would often feel nervous or anxious. I would often have difficulty going shopping, getting headaches, feeling confused and overwhelmed. Often, I would be standing in the checkout line feeling like I wanted to run out of the store. And then, years later, came menopause!

Like most people, I had never given any thought whatsoever to the fact that any of the food I ate or products I used could be harmful or toxic to my family or myself. I believed that if it was advertised, and on the store shelf, then it must be safe to use. I became aware of the fact that fragrance and other common household products made with synthetic petrochemicals had the potential to cause serious adverse side effects in individuals, when I began dating someone who was chemically sensitive. I had to eliminate fragrances, chemicals and mostly everything I had come to use, because it harmed him. I became acutely aware of what a difficult process this can be on a multitude of levels. I found that chemicals and fragrances are found in most every common product. Eliminating them can be frustrating, overwhelming and time consuming.

After I stopped wearing perfume, I also eliminated fragranced soaps and hair care products. I must say that I really had an emotional attachment to certain fragrances. Since eliminating them, I don't miss them at all. I feel much better as a result, and I am quite aware that I do not feel well when I am exposed to them. I immediately get a headache, and feel agitated and anxious, and often dizzy. Funny, those symptoms were often present throughout my life and I did not ever consider that fragrance exposure may be part of the problem.

My skepticism that you could get sick from commonly used products, turned to belief. In 2009, I experienced a chemical injury at work due to faulty ventilation and over exposure to other chemicals. My frustration grew as I experienced not only a variety of adverse physical and emotional symptoms, but was also met by skepticism from the medical community, and others in my life during that time.

There has got to be a better way.
We *can* take control of our health!

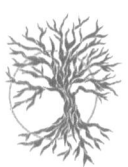

There is another way! You will discover that path as you read the following pages. It's not just empty advice, I also make the best effort to practice what I preach. In the past, I suffered with depression, anxiety, brain fog, and a myriad of other physical problems. I am now on the path to a more informed and mindful lifestyle, and enjoy a healthier life as a result.

I am writing this book because it is my passion to help people understand you can take control of your health.

Sometimes it isn't the barrage of facts and information that inspires people to make changes; sometimes it's by putting a human face on the problem. Sometimes we hear a story and relate to it and that's what makes the difference.

While completing my Master's Degree in Mental Health Counseling in 2011, I conducted and wrote a qualitative narrative research project entitled, "Understanding the Impact of Culturally Prominent Chemicals and Toxins on the Human Mind and Body." I wanted to explore this topic further, not only because of my own personal experience, but also, to listen and learn from the experiences of others.

The following stories are a brief account of seven peoples' struggle through illness to better health. These individuals share stories of how culturally prominent chemicals and toxins affected them, and how their healthy improved when exposure to these substances was limited or eliminated. The people in this study describe common symptoms that send people seeking help to medical offices and mental health practices across the country. These seven-people opted to heal themselves by avoiding toxins. You will learn what motivated these men and women to choose such radical life change, what that process was like, as well as the results from that change.

Much of this book was taken from that project, and revised with current information. I wrote this book with the hope that you could not only understand the experiences of people who struggled with physical and emotional symptoms, but also provide you with research and literature review. Scientific inquiry and literature are vital in understanding that choosing to live "green" is not just a popular phase, political issue or opinion but a matter of health. These people have discovered a path to a healthier life.

I invite you to consider as you read their stories:
Does anything sound familiar in your life?

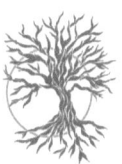

CHAPTER 2
THEIR STORIES

The following seven interviews took place during the month of August 2011. Their names have been changed to honor their privacy. These are people who volunteered for this study and come from all walks of life. The stories of Penny and Wheeler focus on the elimination of fragranced products and complaints of asthma and related symptoms. Two more adults, Allan and Rose, suffered from a cluster of symptoms commonly known as Multiple Chemical Sensitivity. Rose also had other health issues as well. Among the products they eliminated were those containing petrochemicals and synthetic fragrances. Rose also changed her diet to eliminate gluten.

Allan had already eliminated MSG and preservatives early on in his life, as he discovered that it caused feelings of anger and aggression.

Considering increasing rates of Autism, ADHD, ODD and other behavioral issues in children, of particular interest are the stories of Helen, Heather and Alan as they tell how food additives, preservatives and, in one case, fragrance affected the behavior of their children. When these products were eliminated from their diets and households, these parents saw a marked improvement in their children's behavior.

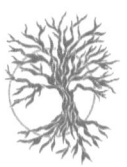

ALAN

I met with Alan at his home. He is a professional musician and teacher and works in the human services field, assisting people with developmental disabilities. He had been diagnosed with Multiple Chemical Sensitivity (MCS) over 20 years ago, resulting in a chemical exposure in a school building where he worked. After a long journey with his illness, he enjoys much improved health now, and chooses to live as toxin free as possible. For Allan, it's absolutely no petrochemicals, synthetic fragrances, or MSG. Allan describes his experience, before eliminating these products, as follows:

"I was a single parent, constantly on the go. I had chronic headaches, consistent anxiety, and depression. I wasn't self-aware, I was much more reactive. I thought I could go anywhere! I never saw the world as a limiting place. Then I started discovering that certain things were making me sick."

For Allen, his current "green lifestyle" was not a choice but a process. "The levels of anxiety and depression I had were unbearable. Anti-depressants made it worse. On Zoloft, I had self-abusive suicidal thoughts that I never had prior. My ability to function diminished. I had headaches all the time. The doctors couldn't help. I was finally given information by someone else who had been chemically injured."

"It was an arduous process. I had no good information at one time; it was all a piecemeal process. I had no idea how insidious it was and that labels didn't mean much. It was a three to four-year process to learn everything I needed to learn. It was a different time (back then). Washington Toxics Coalition was my lifesaver. They gave me access to a doctor who knew something about Environmental Illness. The medical profession was not only useless but invalidating. They had no information on environmental issues or products. They would just give me psychiatric drugs, which almost killed me."

The products Alan stopped using were all petrochemical products, synthetic cleaning fluids, and synthetic fragrances. He had already stopped MSG and additives in his twenties, because he realized he became angry or agitated when he ate them. With MCS, "I eliminated all petrochemical products. I went from Suave to Avalon products, Ivory soap to Kirks, Arm and Hammer to Ecover. I eliminated shaving cream. I eliminated Mop and Glow, Liquid Gold, shower cleaners, Comet, Ajax, Windex and carpet cleaners. I replaced them (all) with vinegar, baking soda, and borax."

Alan describes his health now as much better. "As my system cleared out, and I was no longer constantly surrounded by toxins and chemical load, I was able to distinguish [how I was really feeling and what was the cause]. Prior to that I couldn't tell the difference. I didn't know what

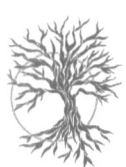

healthy felt like until I was cleared out of all this stuff [chemicals].   Depression, anxiety, vertigo, shakes and tremors, anger and confusion have been eliminated. Headaches only occur about three percent of the time now. I have some seasonal depression still or situational "sadness" or anxiety.

Before traveling to California to learn a new process of healing and recovery from MCS, if I was exposed to products, I would experience symptoms all over again- like if I went to someone's house with Yankee candles, fragrances, colognes or perfumes. It is a matter of degree.   The new process is the weeklong workshop I attended about how to rewire the brain from trauma.   It's foundation is in all the research on the neuroplasticity of the brain.

Alan's story of other people's reactions is similar to others interviewed as he stated; "After being diagnosed with MCS, I found it impossible to live in this culture. I was a pain in the ass to people. I felt like I was a leper. It was the most isolating thing I ever endured. I kept getting told I was crazy, and I believed it! I had enormous difficulty finding a place to work. I lost friends. It was hard to go out in public. I'd either have to leave or get sick."

Alan has never had anyone complain about his use of other products, nor heard complaints about his cleanliness. He has had complaints from others about his need to have them (others) use different products.   His family was extremely resistant. "They don't believe this sort of thing."

Allan wanted to share the following comments for this research:

"I had gone to multiple therapists, due to depression. Only one had any understanding that environmental issues affect mental health. All others were useless, with no benefit as far as helping me with symptoms. I was so sick then; I didn't know. I think a lot of mental illness is environmentally induced, no question. Doctors need to wake up. A drug is not the answer to everything. They have to find causation-an effort to find the question why [sickness or symptoms are happening].

"As far as all the knowledge out there now, I have mixed emotions; I am eternally grateful that there is more info than there was. It's frustrating to watch large corporations being able to continue to lie pathologically about their products. It's uncomfortable to watch the government claim to have an interest in protecting us, when they have only banned four chemicals." "The FDA is protecting the people that they are supposed to be protecting us from. It's frustrating that institutions still have no interest in making changes, despite evidence to the contrary that their stuff is bad. The burden is on the public to prove a product is harmful, instead of companies proving a product is harmless. With the increasing rates of petrochemicals used, there was also increasing rates of cancer and illness."

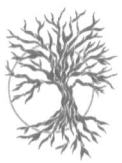

PENNY

It was a warm August afternoon as Penny and I met at a local café after her shift at work. Penny is in her 50's and holds a Master's Degree. She works in upper management in a human services agency. Penny was eager to participate in the interview and share her story.

"Anything I can do to help spread the word."

Penny suffers from asthma and has a serious allergy to fragrance. When recalling her life, prior to going fragrance free, she recalled: "Over time I was bothered by things. Animal dander, then more things began to be a trigger; cigarette smoke, fragrances. I developed asthma. I began to have increasing awareness of headaches, asthma, itchy eyes."

I asked her about her motivation to change and eliminate fragrances from her life. "I wanted to breathe! Fragrances were making me sick! Fragrances contributed to my asthma, headaches and anxiety."

When discussing the difficulty and prominence of fragrances, she reported, "I discovered that fragrance was in everything-shampoos, conditioners, laundry products, and soap."

Penny now uses strictly unscented products. For Penny, the process of switching products was not easy. "Trial and error; I didn't know what to use. I had to try and see. It was frustrating and expensive. Fragrance is part of the culture. People love to cover body odor with fragrance. Some people were tolerant, some didn't want to pay attention. It means people have to make a change."

Penny said that the negative ramifications of going unscented were the cost of products and resentment from others. She sensed an attitude of, 'I don't want to accommodate you', when family members visited.

"When mom is visiting me, she uses soap that isn't fragrance free. It causes an issue and make me sick. My mother would say, 'It's just a little bit.' People don't understand the degree. If they don't smell it, they don't get it. You always hear, 'I just used a little.'"

Penny said that her asthma is gone, since switching to fragrance free, and she is breathing clearer. However, one new problem is that she now has anxiety over being exposed to fragrances. Penny stated that she often must choose between going somewhere to a great event or staying home and remaining healthy. "I'm just not being able to go places for fear that I will run into people wearing fragrance. Sometimes I just stay home."

When asked if she had any additional comments to include in this research she said:

"It's about accommodating disabilities. Some are accommodated, some are not. Where are people's attachments? People think that no fragrance is a preference, not a need! It's a dilemma. [There are] constant decisions

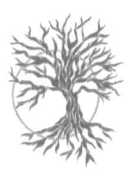

about what to do when exposed - in the workplace, in meetings, etc. Do I stay or do I leave? Maybe people aren't exposed to problems now, but people have to pay attention sooner or later!"

RUTH

Ruth is in her sixties, an advocate and business owner from California. We corresponded via email and set up a time to conduct our interview via telephone. I met Ruth through her website, which sells natural products and provides information for those suffering from Multiple Chemical Sensitivity (MCS). Through her thick English accent, she recounted:

"I had over 14 symptoms, including asthma migraines, allergies, disorientation, dizziness, agitation." Ruth had been everywhere seeking help, but found no improvement. "I was about to die! Finally, I went to a "quack." He said "no gluten, no grains, no sugar, no processed food." I got fifty percent better. So, then I went further. I eliminated dairy, bread, processed meat, coffee, diet drinks, fragrances and perfume. I went to baking soda, Borax and Bon Ami for cleaners."

For her, making the switch was no problem. "This was 25 years ago! I mostly used fragrance-free soap and detergents. I never used makeup or hair dyes, and I never polished my furniture either!" Ruth said that because of these changes, "My MCS was eliminated, and everything else is much less. I still have some joint pain, but no asthma for

25 years and no more migraines! Fibromyalgia was reduced and, if I stopped caffeine, I may get rid of joint pain, but I have chronic fatigue so I'm stuck with it."   Ruth said she did develop low thyroid recently.

No one complained about her use of different products, but as far as a supportive response from others, it was not the case. "No! I lost all my friends, and family, because I couldn't have fragrances in the house. I had even bought someone some soap and asked them that if they were coming to visit me, would they please use this instead. They thought I was crazy! 'How dare you tell me what to wear!"'

Ruth wanted to be sure that her following suggestion was included in this study: "Stop gluten; it stops depression! Food is major. We need vitamin D, pro-biotics, B6. Keep a food diary! You can tell if you go off gluten for three weeks. You can see a difference in four days. No milk, no gluten. Green vegetables. Eat three fruits a day. No sugar. Eat steak or eggs for proteins. Brown rice. Stay away from fluoride!"

WHEELER

Wheeler is a married woman in her fifties. She is a musician, teacher, mother and grandmother. She too has had her own significant health issues, and her contribution to this research focuses on getting rid of fragrances and other toxins.

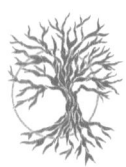

"In my own home, I have had many breathing issues (asthma, asthmatic bronchitis, pneumonia) due to fragrance and strong smells, such as shellac. I decided to cut out as many as I could that were in my control." She switched to unscented products because, "One of my husband's grandsons also has major allergy/breathing issues. I thought that it would also help him when he visited." She eliminated "scented anything, candles, dish detergent, laundry products." Since eliminating fragrances, she found "the difference has been very helpful for me. Wheezing, coughing, watery eyes, hoarseness, have been reduced, and I have fewer serious asthma attacks. I use my Epi pen less frequently, and – at least in my own space – have some control.

The school that I work in has been very aware of my issues, (since I went to the hospital) because they painted my room on a Sunday. I have a severe latex allergy. Once latex paint has "cured", it is fine, but that takes several days. Latex and strong fume issue is a recipe for a trip to the hospital. Last year I broke three ribs from coughing. This turned into asthmatic bronchitis from a bouquet of strong flowers that a school person did not want to remove from the teachers' lounge. I no longer work in that school!"

There was extra benefit of the switch. As for her husband, "I didn't realize that these things were issues for him, but he feels better and has less congestion since we switched out everything three years ago."

The down side for them occurs when their son comes home. "He brings scented products and cologne. It is very tough for the short time he visits."

Wheeler's additional comments that she wanted to share as part of this research: "After suggesting that the grandson might benefit from less chemical fragrance in his home (scented candles everywhere!!!), I am happy to say that his daughter-in-law has cut back and gone to unscented laundry products. I hope there will be some improvement for him also."

The following three stories from parents recount behavior, or behavior and health issues, seen with their sons or daughters.

PETER

The first woman is Helen, who is from Pennsylvania. She completed the survey ahead of time, and we followed up via telephone. Her story is about her son, Peter. He is grown and moved out of the house, but she recounts this experience from when he lived at home. Helen had made the choice to eliminate food additives (colors and flavors) from their diet, after witnessing Pete's behavior,

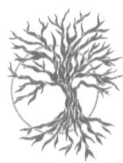

"Peter has not ever made a conscious choice to be chemically free. However, I could identify periods of time when food additives and preservatives were affecting his behavior. He became nasty and much more hyperactive than usual. His perceptions became skewed. I noticed that when he ate artificial additives, his behavior changed. His behavior also was affected by ingesting sugar. Without artificial additives/preservatives (and sugar), Peter correctly perceives other people's actions and appropriately interacts with people. His hyperactivity is greatly reduced.

When Helen decided to change their diet, "I became a label reader. Nothing went into the cart until I knew it was without artificial ingredients. Shopping trips were much longer until I knew what I could purchase. Eating away from home was difficult because, obviously, everyone did not eat this way. Birthday parties at school and friends' homes were special challenges, not only for the additives, but for the sugar. Some people thought I was making a big deal over nothing." When my son's behavior changed from sweet and loving to mean and belligerent, he did not recognize it. So, he did not understand the need to limit and omit some foods."

"When Peter lived with me, we all ate the same way. As long as the meals tasted good and there were tasty snacks available, no one complained." Helen further stated, "I would add a few points: Peter has been diagnosed with bipolar disorder. It is difficult to determine if the additives make his condition worse or if they, on their own, cause his behavioral problems. Peter also has an allergy to aspirin. It causes soft-tissue swelling. Switching to Tylenol is usually an acceptable replacement. Occasionally, foods have also caused this soft-tissue swelling. His tongue swelled from aspartame in gum. Once, oysters caused the problem. Since that appeared only once, perhaps what the oysters ate was the real problem."

KAREN

Heather is a practitioner of alternative medicine in Northern New Hampshire. She describes her daughter as having "frenetic behavior outbursts, where she would move her physical body rapidly and into unusual and sometimes dangerous situations, like climbing a tree with a knife. She was only 8 years old when I noticed she would get out of control after ingesting certain foods or being exposed to other toxins such as fragrances."

Heather's motivating factor was to eliminate "all perfumes and products with perfumes or fragrances-like hair and laundry products - and find "chem free" or organic products" because her daughter's health was at risk. She attributed her daughter's "frenetic behavior and underlying thyroid issue" to the following products, which she eliminated: "any laundry or health & beauty product which has a fragrance in it; fluoride toothpaste; harsh cleaning products like Lysol or Febreze or Glade air fresheners; all

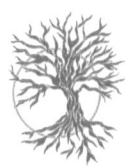

ramen noodles; canned soup; taco seasoning and chips with MSG; many drinks with artificial colors and ingredients."

Heather describes the process as: "It took time to evaluate all the labels, and we had to read everything, including all food products which may have contained MSG and its subsequent pen names. I was often worried that the label didn't tell honestly what was in it.

The search was difficult until our grocery store added an organic section, which made it a bit easier. Even though the prices may have seemed higher at first, they last longer and we were better nourished by it. As a result, we feel more energized and feel better overall by eating healthy foods and keeping harsh chemicals out of our home environment"

Heather says there have been no complaints about her switching, but states, "No complaints, only judgments about it, as if I were silly and making it all up, because why would a corporation sell us something that may cause us harm? My children, ages 8 & 13 at the time, were supportive. My ex-husband was resistant, and still has a level of disbelief and non-compliance even though our daughter became, and has remained, healthy as a result of this removal."

MIKE

Allan tells of the effect that food additives and preservatives had on his son, Mike. "Mike was hyperactive and agitated. He had no peripheral vision, meaning he would not take into consideration or notice things around him. He was aggressive."

There wasn't necessarily a motivating factor but a significant event that caused Allan to rid artificial flavors and colors from Mike's diet. "I was watching him play pee wee football, and saw him eat skittles on the sidelines, and watched him turn into a terror on the field. It was like a drug with him. [He had] no ability to be thoughtful. I knew MSG was an issue with me, but then I saw it in him, especially the artificial colors. The specific things that Allan eliminated were "any type of candy with colors, which is most of them. I pushed fruit and chocolate. I made my own soups instead of Campbell's, no packaged foods, potatoes instead of tater-tots. I read the ingredients in salad dressings."

"I was already a label reader, due to not using MSG. The difficulty was that anywhere else he went, he would eat it, because he was in denial. Food at school is loaded [with additives and preservatives]! Soups, jello, etc. In the beginning, it was hard because I had to educate myself. I stopped wasting time in the candy aisle. I learned which companies were safe. I was still unaware of hidden things on labels, and not aware of how they disguised food. I shopped the produce, meat and dairy aisles of the store."

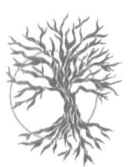

I asked Allan if there were any issues related to making the change. "The only negative thing from switching [to healthier products] was the stress of knowing that I could not do anything about what he did when he left the house. When he ate that crap, he was more likely to get into trouble. Angry kids lead to aggressive behavior."

As far as people's reactions, "parents considered it a nuisance. Schools will not look at anything. They only respond when required to do so by law. They didn't even investigate the possibility that it was an issue."

Allan described what it was like when Mike did not have any food additives. "It was immediate, one hour after eating, like flipping the switch. On it, you got aggression, ADD, ODD. He was a different person when not eating additives. He was sensitive, perceptive, kind, and genuine; he was a decent kid. When he ate it he was belligerent and uncontrollable. The only thing remaining was his difficulty concentrating. I think he had that in general. But usually I saw an immediate change in him within one hour after eating.

It's hard to say what Mike's overall health is today. "He didn't stay with it, [there was] gross inconsistency in his life; [he had] constant exposure to chemicals; he didn't believe [their negative impact] and was often in an agitated state. He was unable to process emotionally, got pissed off, and easily fell into drugs. He ended up in long-term trouble." Allan's additional comments for the research were: "On the flip side of aggression, was depression. Inside of an hour he would be wound up and pissed off. The more he ate it, the more he wanted. Also, sending him to school with lunch from home was ostracizing, so at school he got school lunch, complete with artificial colors, flavors and MSG."

AND OTHERS

While hanging a flyer to recruit research participants in a local community center, one woman wanted to share her son's story, but didn't have time to do an interview. Georgia is a young woman in her thirties with a son in elementary school. She talked about how she discovered that the sun screen she and her husband had been using on him was making him very ill. She recalled that soon after she had used the sunscreen, her son would become lethargic, and then spike a fever, often as high as 105.

"It was after the third time he got sick that we finally figured out what was happening! The doctors didn't even know what was wrong."

She also had been experiencing increasing skin rashes, which she finally traced to soaps, shampoos and laundry products. Dermatologists had not helped.

"I am now in the process of trying to switch to natural products with cleaners and laundry soaps, fragrance free, etc., but it's actually overwhelming. I had to stop for a while. I was getting paranoid, and everything has something in it! I figured if they sold it in the stores, it was safe."

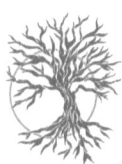

CHAPTER 3
COMMON THREADS

I want to express my gratitude to the wonderful people who were willing to share their stories for this project. For some it was a sensitive issue, and yet they were happy to have someone that was interested in their story, especially from the field of mental health or what was considered traditional practice. I was apprehensive at first, but I was greeted with openness and "I'm very happy to help spread the news" responses. Some of these folks needed care and compassion as some relived the distress and grief of their experiences. Many endured great loss - anywhere from loss of career, loss of freedom to do things they enjoy, losing friends, family and relationships, and the disbelief and non-cooperation of family members in relation to their health issues. Many were told they were crazy by family and professionals.

There was also considerable frustration on the part of parents, who realized that certain foods their children had been eating had been making them sick or contributing to emotional and behavioral problems. Common in the process was the frustration of finding healthy alternatives and realizing how many labels often mislead or omit harmful ingredients.

After each interview, I began to see the common threads weaving their experiences together. It seemed as though each of these individuals chose to eliminate common products in favor of organic, fragrance-free and natural products. This choice stemmed from either a serious health issue or an emotional or behavioral issue resulting from the use, or exposure, to common everyday products sold on the store shelves.

I was struck by two things in particular: the disillusionment over the fact that they thought that products sold in the stores were safe; and that labels often didn't tell the whole story. Their health issues and resulting choices were often very isolating when it came to the need to eliminate fragrance.

People are often uncooperative, dismissing and not accommodating when it comes to not being able to wear or use fragrance around someone who is adversely affected. People with obvious disabilities are often more easily

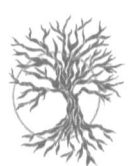

understood and accommodated. The fragrance issue is something that we are still a long way from dealing with. It is in fact worse - with air fresheners and odorizers everywhere you go. More awareness, education, and acceptance that this is a problem, is needed.

The one limitation I faced was that due to time factors, this study was limited to seven people during a single semester at graduate school. However, it is an accurate account of seven people who chose to be part of this project.

I found some common threads from their stories. Each person answered the same twelve questions that focused on basic areas such as: a description of their life and symptoms before eliminating toxins; the reasons why they decided to switch to organic and healthy products; what that process was like; what, if any, symptoms were eliminated; and what were other people's reactions to them as a result of needing to make this change.

The common motivating factors for people reducing or eliminating exposure to toxins were: health risks; being sick; experiencing or witnessing emotional and/or behavior problems in themselves or their children. Exposure to toxins contributed to symptoms that affected the respiratory, auto immune, neurological and behavioral systems.

FOOD ADDITIVES

Certain themes began to emerge as I tallied up symptoms and problems that had been mentioned. Each time a separate trait or symptom was mentioned, I counted it as a single occurrence.

The following is a relationship of adverse reactions reported when food additives and preservatives were ingested.

- ADHD or hyperactivity are the behaviors described as such, were reported three times.

- Behavioral Problems are described as out of control, defiant, or dangerous/impulsive behaviors; those were reported four times.

- Anger and aggression were reported five times.

- Perceptions (unable to perceive others correctly) were reported twice.

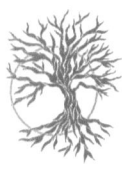

FRAGRANCE

Certain themes began to emerge as I tallied up symptoms and problems that had been mentioned. Each time a separate trait or symptom was mentioned, I counted it as a single occurrence.

The following is a relationship of adverse reactions reported when there was an exposure to fragrances.

- Respiratory problems: asthma; asthmatic bronchitis; pneumonia and allergies; reported seven times.

- Various neurological symptoms were described such as: headaches; migraines; disorientation; dizziness; agitation; depression and anxiety; reported ten times

- Auto Immune covering: Multiple Chemical Sensitivity; Chronic Fatigue; and Fibromyalgia and thyroid problems; reported five times.

- Behavioral, out of control, defiant or dangerous/impulsive behaviors; reported twice.

I often heard that the medical and mental health professions had not been helpful. As a last resort, individuals found solutions by trial and error themselves or by going to alternative health professionals. As Penny stated,

"I finally went to a quack!".

Some found doctors who specialized in environmental medicine. Professionals in the main stream never questioned the food or products they were using.   People often felt discounted, and spent a lot of time and money on tests with no improvement or, as in the case of Alan, prescribed anti-depressants that caused more harm.

Once individuals discovered that products such as fragrance, common household cleaners, food additives and preservatives were causing their symptoms, they took charge of their own health and began the process of researching what were healthy and safe alternatives.

When the exposure to the offending substance was stopped, symptoms were either eliminated or significantly reduced.

There was also an improvement in behavior, such as a decrease in aggression, impulsive behavior, anger, or lack of interpersonal awareness.

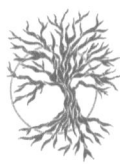

There was a common assumption, from most, that products on the store shelves were safe. The process to eliminate toxins was often overwhelming as more time was spent reading labels.

As one mom put it, "I didn't put anything in my cart unless I read the label."

Another realization was that certain toxins, such as food additives, preservatives and fragrances, were everywhere!

Sadly, making these changes came at a cost. Support from family and friends was not consistent with participants. Wheeler's husband benefited health-wise, as well as his grandson, from eliminating fragrance from the home.

Food can be a particular issue, as eliminating "junk food" from kids' diets can be challenging. When kids go out to school or to friends' homes, often they are exposed to delicious toxic treats. Others found that even family members can sabotage the food issue by not attending to a particular diet and by their own disbelief that food additives and preservatives are a problem.

Some family members, especially surrounding the fragrance or chemical issue, were disbelieving. It also was evident that some family members still chose to wear or bring fragrance into the home of the person it made sick. This poses not only physical difficulty but emotional stress and anxiety as well. Why do people disregard or disbelieve this issue?

Penny's statement explains it when she said, "It's about accommodating disabilities – some (people) are accommodating, some are not. Where are people's attachments? People think that no fragrance is a preference, not a need! It's a dilemma."

Do you recognize yourself or a family member in these stories? Does their experience sound familiar?

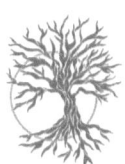

CHAPTER 4
WHAT WE DON'T KNOW *CAN* HURT US!

When people seek help from traditional medical and mental health practices, often missing from the equation is a deeper assessment lifestyle habits. Typical questions ask about caffeine, tobacco, alcohol/drug use, sleep and exercise patterns. What's missing, is to consider how the quality of food people eat and what kind of products people use could be impacting the person's health and wellbeing.

How can that be accomplished in what the current system allows in a 15-minute appointment with your PCP, or the traditional intake assessment in a mental health facility?

It cannot.

In conversations, I've had with people throughout the years, I find a common thread with lifestyle habits. I also hear people wondering why they are still sick, despite all their medications. Let me state that I am not blaming or judging here - these are only observations. As a matter of fact, I used to have some of these same habits!

These common habits are socially acceptable, heavily advertised and promoted in our culture.

Consumption or use of:
- soda, diet soda, fast foods, processed foods, non-organic, GMO foods,
- use of common health and beauty products,
- use of deodorizers/air fresheners in their homes and automobiles,
- use and exposure to scented candles and heavily scented, petroleum based laundry and cleaning products with common household cleaning products, pesticides and plastics.

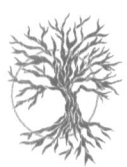

The organic and green lifestyle has grown in popularity over the years, yet the average person has limited knowledge regarding the dangers of toxins and chemicals lurking in common products found on our grocery store shelves. In fact, since World War II, ten thousand plus chemicals have been introduced into our environment. Only ten percent of these chemicals have been tested at all. None have been tested for long term, low level exposure.

We trust product labels, which can often omit ingredients or mislead us into thinking that what we are buying is safe and healthy. These common products are heavily promoted, advertised and socially acceptable. It's a deeply ingrained yet societal myth that the products and food sold to us are safe. So why should we stop and worry about it. Just one more thing on the stack of the hundreds of other concerns in our worlds!

I find this a hard topic to discuss with people. I'm often met with resistance or denial. This is due to something called *cognitive dissonance.* In psychology, cognitive dissonance is described as: the stress and discomfort experienced by a person when they are confronted by new information that conflicts with existing beliefs or values; holds two or more contradictory beliefs or values at the same time; or performs an action that is contradictory to their beliefs or values. For example; When I became aware that I had spent most my life using and exposing my family to harmful products, I was in denial, then shock, enraged then paranoid. Our world can suddenly seem very hazardous and frightening if we acknowledge that our belief in corporations, companies and stores (who would not sell things to us if they were not safe), is a common societal myth and,

A Lie!

Despite the increasing amount of scientific research in recent years concerning the effects of toxins on individuals (especially in relation to children and learning disabilities), little of this research has found its way into the everyday lives of people. Regardless of the mounting evidence linking disease and these chemical exposures, there is a rising epidemic of diseases, learning disabilities, cancers and mental health issues.

Most practitioners in the fields of traditional medicine and mental health are often unaware of the dangers and health implications of toxins found in the common products and foods. This information exists in environmental and alternative medicine; however, it is not typically addressed in traditional medical training. It's not even part of treatment protocol. It was not part of my curriculum for my degree in mental health counseling. So, unless a provider is personally aware of the links between chemicals, toxins and illness, it won't be discussed or considered.

I believe that this is due to a lack of training & education, not a lack of care.

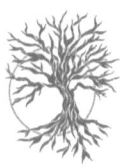

Consider: Perhaps this absence of information has something to do with the heavy promotion, influence, and money of Big Pharma; as there is indeed a prescription for everything that ails us.

I believe, for the most part, that people try to do the best they can. Most, try to improve their life - whether it be starting a new fitness program, taking vitamins and supplements, practicing yoga/meditation, deepening a spiritual practice, choosing to begin therapy to resolve current or past issues, or improve relationships. All those things are all wonderful and beneficial.

The truth is that if we continue to dump toxins in our body, it's pretty much all for naught.

I truly believe from the research and my own personal experience, true health and wellness is only possible when, in addition to those things, we eliminate toxins from our food and products as much as possible.

I now see with clients in Private Practice. I started Eden Living because I believe in a holistic approach of mind, body and spirit. Eden Living represents a lifestyle approach to emotional wellness, which blends mindfulness practice, education and awareness about how taking care of our bodies (especially the food we eat and the products we use) can affect our wellbeing, and the importance of spiritual practice for optimal wellbeing. I believe wellness attends to all three.

If you are serious about your health (and I know you are if you are reading this book) tired of suffering, or you a person able to make an impact in the lives of other people, I encourage you to keep an open and curious mind about how reducing or eliminating toxins and chemicals from your food, homes and personal care products, is a key foundation to good health. When you do this, all the other healthy changes in your life will have a greater and more lasting impact.

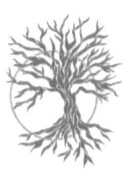

"IT IS NO MEASURE OF HEALTH TO BE WELL ADJUSTED

TO A PROFOUNDLY SICK SOCIETY." KRISHNAMURTI:

CHAPTER 5
A SYSTEM IN CRISIS

I began my counseling career in a community mental health setting, where individuals identified as having severe and persistent mental illness could receive services. During my time there, I was blessed to have the opportunity to have a wonderful supervisor, and work with some great people. I finally left my position because frankly, I could no longer handle the stress and frustration of working in a system whose model is "broken, failing and in crisis". I am not alone in that assessment. In 2011, the US Department of Justice Civil Rights Division called New Hampshire's mental system exactly that. The mental health system in the United States received a D from The National Alliance on Mental Illness (NAMI) in 2009. By the time I left, it wasn't faring any better.

My colleges and I worked with dedication and perseverance, despite severely limited-to-no resources. My frustration and despair grew as I watched clients, adults and children, who desperately needed hospitalization, spend days in an ER waiting for a bed that was not available, or just sent back home to "wait it out". This was often the norm, not the exception. Those seeking mental health services, either spend months, not days, waiting for an intake appointment, or they get referred to another facility, because the waiting list is months out. Often, existing caseloads are so unmanageable, that the prescribers and/or therapists can no longer accept any new clients, and they can barely keep up with the existing paperwork and productivity requirements.

Those working in the system and the individuals and their loved ones seeking services are desperate. The result of this broken and failing system, is that a client's symptoms become more severe, resulting in a myriad of serious consequences.

Once in the "system", in the current American model, clients often go through trial and error of finding the right medication while enduring serious and sometimes debilitating side effects. They may be labeled as "resistant" or "non-compliant" for not wanting to take their medications. These medications often carry a lifetime sentence.

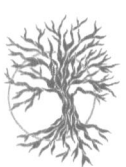

Finland, takes an opposite approach, that we would benefit by adopting in this country. In 1980, Finland pioneered the "open dialogue" model, which looks at the interrelation of social factors in a person's life, (not just symptoms) and utilizes a team approach, including client, family and providers in treatment. This results in reducing the need for medication and hospitalization for people experiencing first episode psychosis. (Carter 2015).

Add to the US crisis, in the world outside community mental health, individuals, referred to as the "worried well", often seek help through their primary care doctors or other private practice prescribers. Consider the following information from the CDC on some of the most commonly prescribed medications.

- anti-depressant use has increased 400% in the last decade. (CDC, 2011)
- Between 1996 and 2013, anti-anxiety medications, (Benzodiazepines) increased 67% from 8.1 to 13.5 million Americans. (Bachuber, 2016)
- 5,500 people start to use prescription pain medication every day. Often people are taking more than just pain meds. (CDC)
- Overdoses involving pain meds kill more people than coke and heroin combined, and in 2011, 31 percent of those deaths, benzodiazepines were involved. (CDC)

I began to look at the current trends in prescription use and the money and influence of "Big Pharma". Billions of dollars are spent on promoting and advertising their drugs. Realize, that psychiatric medications are a multibillion dollar business. For example, medications for ADHD alone reached $12.9 billion in sales by 2015. It is projected to hit the 17.5-billion-dollar mark, by 2020 making it the top pharmaceutical on the market. (Whelan 2015).

Big Pharma guarantees the public that there is a pill
to cure or at least cope with the consequences
of living in an often emotionally and physically toxic society.

In addition, DSM 5, (which is the manual to diagnose mental disorders) feeds this cycle by often mislabeling normal human life experiences into major mental disorders. Sadly, often overlooked, is a potential underlying medical, physical or social cause to the symptoms of "depression" or "anxiety" that could be relieved by simple diet, supplement or lifestyle change. Instead, often we seek a "pill to quickly cure what ails us" because that's what we have been programed to do. It's easy, isn't it? I know it was for me.

First, let me say that this is not about pointing fingers. If you are someone who takes these medications or prescribes them, (or both for that matter),

I'm not judging you.

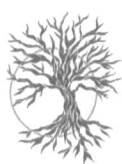

It's the system. We do what we have been programed to do. We go to our health care provider armed with the latest information we found on Google, reinforced by that lovely woman in the TV add, who took that pill and now lives a happily-ever-after life. I'm not saying that all prescription medications are bad. They have their place. I'm asking that we be informed, take a step back and consider, before we take that pill, if there may be another option we haven't considered.

In 2008, an article was published in a Canadian Journal reflecting the crisis in their health care system.

> *...the contemporary model of evidence-based medicine has not effectively addressed the public health dilemma of escalating chronic illness, and there is pervasive dissatisfaction among both patients and caregivers. There is deteriorating morale within the medical community, and unprecedented numbers of discontented patients are turning to assorted unconventional therapies in search of help (Genuis, 2008).*

Research shows that mental health issues are common throughout the United States, affecting tens of millions (1 in 5) people each year. (CDC 2008). The following statistics on reported cases, are from the National Institute of Mental Health.

ADULTS
Age 18 and up

An average of 1 in 4 adults suffer from a diagnosable mental disorder in a given year.

In 2014, there were an estimated 43.6 million adults in the United States, aged 18 or older, with a mental illness. This number represented 18.1% of all U.S. adults. Of these, 9.8 million qualified as severe mental illness. This number represented 4.2% of all U.S. adults.

Approximately 18.1 % of the population has an anxiety disorder in a given year, with an onset at 11 years old. Anxiety disorders include: general anxiety; post-traumatic stress disorder; obsessive-compulsive disorder; and specific phobias, to name a few. Collectively, they are among the most common mental disorders experienced by Americans

9.5 % of the population will suffer from a mood disorder/depressive illness in a given year. This category represents an underlying problem that primarily affects a person's persistent emotional state (their mood).

In 2015, an estimated 16.1 million adults in the United States had at least one major depressive episode in the past year. This number represented 6.7% of all U.S. adults. Bipolar disorder represents 2.6 % with an average onset of age 20.

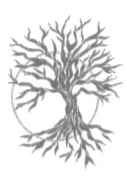

CHILDREN
Age 13 – 17

Unfortunately, mental disorders are common among children in the United States. Just over 20 percent (or 1 in 5) children either currently, or at some point during their life, have had a **seriously** debilitating mental disorder.

Anxiety Disorders in children are found to be 25.1 % with 5.9 % of that considered severe,

14% of children are diagnosed with mood disorders (major depressive disorder, dysthymic disorder, and/or bipolar disorder) with 4.7 % of those considered severe.

In 2015, an estimated 3 million adolescents in the United States, aged 12 to 17, had at least one major depressive episode. This number represented 12.5% children. 2.1 million had at least one major depressive episode with severe impairment. This represents 8.8%

Lifetime prevalence for any diagnosable Mental Disorder in children is 46.3 % with 21.4 % severe.

ADHD diagnosis in children: as of 2012, one in 10 children age 13 – 17 were diagnosed with ADHD – up from 1 in 12 in 2007.

About 1 in 6 children in the United States had a developmental disability in 2006-2008, ranging from mild disabilities, such as speech and language impairments, to serious developmental disabilities such as intellectual disabilities, cerebral palsy, and autism (CDC).

In 2000, Autism rates were 1 in 150. In 2012, it was 1 in 68 children. Autism is 4.5 times more common in boys (1 in 42) than girls (1 in 89).

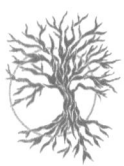

CHRONIC DISEASE

Many individuals I see in my practice also suffer with chronic disease. I was aware that it was prevalent, but I decided to look more closely at the exact numbers. I investigated the National Health Council, CDC, and an article published by Fight Chronic Disease entitled, 'The Growing Crisis of Chronic Disease in the US, and came up with the following disturbing statistics.

Chronic Disease is defined as an ongoing incurable illness or conditions such as heart disease, asthma, cancer and diabetes. The key point is that these diseases are often preventable and frequently manageable with improved lifestyle. The National Health Council and the CDC both report that approximately 133 million Americans, about half the population, have a chronic disease. 8 percent of children (age 5 – 17) are reported by their parents to have limited activities due to at least one chronic disease. Most people have not just one but two or more conditions. Almost a third of the population lives with multiple chronic conditions. In 2009, 7 out of 10 deaths (1.7 million people) were due to chronic disease. It is also estimated that by 2025, chronic disease will affect an estimated 164 million Americans.

Obesity is skyrocketing. According to Business Week, Americans spend 40 billion dollars on weight loss products and programs yet, according to health statistics, we lead the world in obesity and unhealthy lifestyle. It is estimated that approximately 250 million Americans fall into the category of overweight or obese. Childhood obesity rates have tripled since 1980. About 1 in 6 kids (9 million) were overweight in 2004. Given current trends, it is estimated that one in three children born in 2000 will develop diabetes over the course of their lifetime and will most likely be the first generation to have shorter lifespans then their parents.

Think about it: Americans are spending over 40 Billion dollars on weight loss; people with chronic conditions account for 81 % of hospital admissions and 76 % of physician visits; and, get this, 91% of all prescriptions filled! **Think about it:** Who profits from the decline of health of over half the population in this country? These conditions are mostly

PREVENTABLE

The CDC estimates that by simple lifestyle changes we could prevent
80 % of heart disease & stroke
80% of type 2 diabetes
40% of cancers.

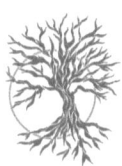

CHAPTER 6
CONSIDER THIS

A little less than half of Americans (45%), actively try to include organic foods in their diets, while 15% actively avoid them. More than a third (38%) say they "don't think either way" about organic foods (Gallup July 2014).

A concerning amount of people still live in a dangerously toxic state and are totally unaware of it. Before that first cup of coffee, about ten personal care products are used each day, and more if you are a woman who uses beauty products. The toothpaste, shampoo, deodorant, baby powder and other products we routinely use expose hundreds of different chemicals.

Many diseases *are* related genetics, diet and lifestyle, but many are also caused by a buildup of toxins that overwhelm the body's systems. Exposure to these toxins produce symptoms such as memory loss, premature aging, skin disorders, arthritis, hormone imbalances, chronic fatigue, anxiety, emotional disorders, cancers, heart disease and many more. Dr. Colbert (2001).

Consider the popularity of the green and organic movements, which have given rise to additional organic and natural sections in the grocery stores, as well as specialty markets such as Whole Foods and other natural food stores and co-ops. Choices for healthy products are more widely available to the consumer, as well as information for recipes to make household cleaners that are cheaper, including often-safer alternatives to other products on the shelves.

Although the organic movement has existed since before the 1940's, there still exists about half the population that downplays or denies the dangerous effects that common products, made with these toxins, have on our bodies. What motivates some individuals that make a switch to an organic, toxic free lifestyle and why do some ignore it? Consider the following quotes from Mt. Sinai and others:

> Over eighty-thousand chemicals have been developed since World War II, and seventy-five percent of the top twenty chemicals that are set into the environment are known or suspected to be toxic to the developing human brain.

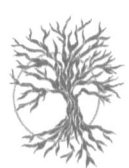

Every year, between 2000 and 3000 new chemicals are registered by the EPA and added to the 75,000 chemicals and millions of mixtures already in use. Most are not carefully studied for health effects and only a handful have been thoroughly evaluated for neurotoxic effects (National Research Council 1992).

The human body deals with toxins by a detox process, disposing of most of them through digestion, elimination, breathing, and sweating. Of the tens of thousands of chemicals, we are exposed to every day, scientists estimate that we carry approximately 700 contaminants in our body. There is a limit to what the body can handle without adverse reactions. Some chemicals cannot be automatically removed from the body and remain in our blood, fat tissue, muscles, bones, brain tissue and other organs. All of these chemicals contribute to our "body burden"- the total amount of chemicals present in our body at one time.

Since we are all unique, each individual can handle body burdens differently. Some bodies can detox better than others and this has to do with genetics. That is why toxins affect some people more than others. (Morrison, 2011).

Scientists have already concluded that fetal and early childhood exposure to industrial chemicals in the environment lead to neurological developmental disorders, autism, attention deficit, and mental retardation. (Toxic Children How US Babies Became Born Pre-polluted).

> In 1987, Autism was estimated to be 1 in 10,000 children. Today it is 1 in 68. (NHMH-NIMH Statistics, 2010)

Childhood cancer is also on the rise, and over 90 percent of all childhood cancers are caused by environmental factors. This means that most of this cancer is preventable. (Imus 2011)

In the report "In Harm's Way", a study conducted by Physicians for Social Responsibility, the following was stated:

> It is estimated that nearly 17 percent of children under 18, in the US, suffer from one or more learning, behavioral or developmental disorders.

> it was shown that these disabilities are clearly the result of complex interactions combining genetics, environmental and social factors during vulnerable periods of development.

> The reason toxic exposure deserves special attention is that it is a preventable cause of harm! (In Harms Way: Toxic Threats to Child Development, 2000).

People suffering from illness and dis-ease are desperate for help and all too often, the root of their issues is unknown. Therapists and health practitioners see individuals with many

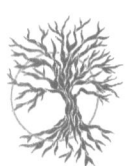

of these symptoms every day. Numerous assessment and screening tools are used to render the appropriate diagnosis. Often these clients are referred to health care providers or psychiatrists, who prescribe medications that, in essence, mask the symptom without getting to the core of the dis-ease. Often these prescriptions create other health problems and side effects, or as some people state, are not really that helpful. There may be a better solution.

We need to move beyond diagnosing symptoms and get to the root of the problem or, in a perfect world, the problems would be prevented in the first place.

We can't solve problems
by using the same kind of thinking
we used when we created them.
Albert Einstein

CONSIDER:

What if some of the food you were eating or products you were using, were contributing to poor physical, emotional or behavioral health?

What if, by making wiser choices, you could can begin to be in control of your health?

What if, by eliminating toxins and making wiser personal choices in the products you use, you could begin to heal your body from dis-ease?

What if, by making healthy choices, you could begin to experience greater physical and mental wellbeing?

IMPORTANT:

**Consult your healthcare provider before you make any changes, especially with prescribed medications.
You could risk serious and/or dangerous side effects.**

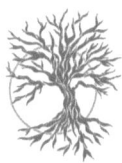

A MISSING LINK

There is a significant body of research among environmental medicine that shows the dangers of environmental toxins and their effects on the human mind and body. There is also a significant number of advocacy websites related to this topic, encouraging and educating consumers on how to make healthier decisions about the products they purchase and food they eat. Although the information is available if one knows where to look, it is strangely absent in the review of literature in mainstream medicine and mental health. This is not a new body of knowledge.

Sickness from toxic exposure in the workplace was not taken seriously until the EPA headquarters building in Washington DC reported hundreds of workers with symptoms of "sick building syndrome" because of remodeling and re-carpeting in the late 80's.

A 1995 issue of Archives of Environmental Health described 75 people who said they became ill following remodeling of their home or workplace, and another 37 said they became ill following a chemical exposure with pesticides. In both groups, exposure to either volatile organic chemicals in the remodeling, or pesticide exposure, was reported with similar symptoms and intolerances. (Miller C.S., 1995).

Behavioral toxicology surfaced as a discipline around 1970. Unfortunately, psychiatry does not often consider toxicology in explaining some behavioral disorders. Neurotoxicity is barely mentioned in psychiatric textbooks, except in instances of gross poisoning in the case of overdosing on medication or substances. Bernard Weiss, (Weiss, 1998) explains that our central nervous system is particularly vulnerable to toxicants. Neurons develop increasingly complex branches over time, while some areas in the brain lose neurons with age.

One aspect that is crucial to our understanding is that brain damage early in life, particularly during fetal and neonatal development, may not emerge until late in life, when the brain's reserve capacity is compromised. This is what is called "silent damage."

It would seem as though health practitioners of various disciplines are on the same playground but are playing in their own sandboxes, unaware of the information and research on the link with health and environmental toxins. Traditional medical and mental health practice needs to bridge the gap between them and other disciplines for a collective body of knowledge that will lead to better overall health and well-being.

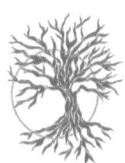

CHAPTER 7

Effect of Toxins on Body Systems

To understand how chemicals and toxins impact the mind and body, we take a closer look at some of the main systems of the body and some common disorders that occur in those systems. When these illnesses are seen through the lens of exposure to environmental toxins, this poses some disturbing questions. This is a cursory review of some of these systems only. Remember biology/physiology:

CENTRAL NERVOUS SYSTEM

The central nervous system is made up of the brain, spinal cord and optic nerve. It controls thought process, movement, and registers sensations in the body. Christopher Reeve Foundation's website puts CNS function eloquently:

"It is the center of our thoughts, interpreter of external environment, and controls body movement."

According to Johns Hopkins, a CNS disorder can affect either the brain or spinal cord, resulting in neurological or psychiatric disorders. The CNS is vulnerable and can be damaged by: trauma, infections, degeneration, autoimmune disorders, structural deficits and stroke.

IMMUNE SYSTEM

Our immune system protects the body from foreign substances and pathogenic organisms. An important part of this system is the lymphatic system. Basically, an autoimmune disorder is when the body attacks and destroys healthy body tissue by mistake. A key component of an auto immune disorder is inflammation. There are more than 80 types of autoimmune disorders, and people can have more than one at a time. Some common autoimmune disorders are: rheumatoid arthritis; lupus; inflammatory bowel disease; multiple sclerosis; Hashimoto's Thyroiditis; type 1 diabetes, cancers and others.

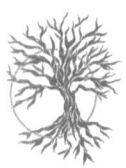

ENDOCRINE SYSTEM

The endocrine system is the collection of glands that produce hormones which regulate metabolism, growth and development, tissue function, sexual function, reproduction, sleep and mood, among other things. The endocrine system is made up of the pituitary gland, thyroid gland, parathyroid glands, adrenal glands, pancreas, ovaries and testicles. It is important because this system affects almost every organ and cell in the body. (Zimmerman, 2016)

RESPIRATORY SYSTEM

The respiratory system is in charge of the intake of oxygen and output of carbon dioxide from the body. Nose, mouth pharynx and larynx bring air into to the lungs. Common Disorders of the respiratory system include: influenza, pneumonia, asthma, and COPD.

Effects of Toxins on Children's Health

Babies are being born polluted. A recent study, conducted by The Environmental Working Group, analyzed umbilical cord blood collected from 10 infants born in 2007 and 2008. The laboratories identified up to 232 industrial compounds and pollutants in these babies. This research demonstrates that industrial chemicals cross the placenta to contaminate a baby before birth.

The contaminants found are some of the most problematic consumer products and commercial chemicals ever put on the market and can be found in any American household. Brominated flame retardants, PCBs, the Teflon chemical PFOA and the Scotchgard chemical PFOS, BPA, lead, mercury, perchlorate, dioxins and furans are all considered either likely human carcinogens, serious neurotoxins, or well-established hormone disrupters, according to government health authorities. (Group, 2009)

A summary of the chemicals found in Environmental Working Groups study is found in Appendix A.

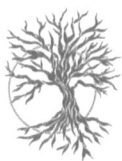

Children are especially vulnerable, and consequences are more severe, when exposed to environmental toxins - with particular attention to four of the most damaging of environmental dangers: (Burstyn & Sampson, 2005)

- persistent organic pollutants (POPs), i.e. pesticides;
- agricultural hormones in the food chain;
- antibiotics in the food chain;
- heavy metals such as mercury and lead.

> Children at different stages of development have unique physical risk factors with different types of exposure. When children are exposed to contaminants, the way in which they absorb, distribute, and metabolize chemicals will affect how their bodies deal with the foreign substance (Bearer, 1995).

Developmental, learning, and behavioral disabilities are a growing health problem. Environmental chemicals interfere with brain development during critical periods, affecting sensory, motor, and cognitive function.

> Because regulation in the United States is based on a proof of harm rather than proof of lack of harm, it is unknown at what exact percentage these chemicals cause problems. The most important point is: the hazards of environmental pollutants are inherently preventable. (Koger, Schettler, & Weiss, 2005)

Neurodevelopment, Behavior and Cognition

Social stress and environmental toxins affect early neurodevelopment. Environmental factors can promote or disrupt this process, depending on whether they are positive (social supports, good nutrition, etc.) or negative (psychosocial stress, chemical toxicants, malnutrition, trauma, etc.) The endpoint appears to be changes in the development and formation of memory.

Acute stress may enhance memory formation, but chronic stress inhibits it. While neuro-plasticity allows recovery from short-term toxic exposures, chronic stress could induce permanent structural or organizational changes (Wright, 2009).

Schettler et al. reports on the contribution of chemical contamination to an epidemic of developmental, learning, and behavioral disabilities affecting America's children today.

> *"Disabilities are clearly the result of complex interactions among genetic, environmental and social factors that impact children during vulnerable periods of development."*

Scientists are focusing on genetic make-up and environmental 'triggers.' Certain genes can increase one's susceptibility to a contaminant by altering metabolism of the contaminant in the body, decreasing (or increasing) one's ability to detoxify a specific contaminant, or causing

68

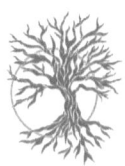

inappropriate immune system reactions to particular compounds. Studies show conclusively that:

"A variety of chemicals commonly encountered in industry and the home can contribute to developmental, learning and behavioral disorders." *"Most people remain ignorant of these findings, including many obstetricians and pediatricians, who should and could be providing solid, responsible advice to parents and parents-to-be on simple steps to reduce risks attributed to childhood behavioral disabilities." (Schettler & Stein, 2000).*

The Developing Brain Is Central To This Issue.

Almost all birth defects involve impaired central nervous system (CNS) functioning. Neurotoxins interfere with various specific developmental (CNS) processes. Any impairment by at least one neurotoxin (lead or methylmercury for example) can lead to scrambled or impaired behavioral function. There are various classes of neurotoxins: heavy metals; polychlorinated biphenyls; pesticides; herbicides; organic solvents; environmental tobacco smoke; radiation and endotoxins. This vast amount of environmental neurotoxins could account for a wide variety of cases of MR currently classified as "due to unknown causes". (Schroeder, 2000).

Even breast milk has been found as a source of toxins! A report from Northwest Environmental Watch showed an analysis of breast milk samples, donated by nine Puget Sound mothers, which revealed high levels of toxic flame retardants in every sample tested. Concentrations of the chemicals were 20 to 40 times the levels found in Europe and Japan.

American residents contain the world's highest concentrations of PBDEs. These toxic compounds are known to cause behavioral aberrations, learning deficits, and other health effects in laboratory animals (Watch, 2004).

The association between environmentally released mercury and special education and autism rates in Texas were investigated. Texas Department of Education and the EPA found that on average for every 1000 lb. of environmentally released mercury there was an increase in special education services by 43 % and autism by 61% (Palmer, Blanchad, Stein, Mandell, & Miller, 2006).

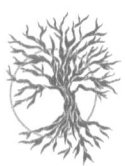

ILLNESS THOUGH A DIFFERENT LENS

In the chapters that follow, you will see how different chemicals and toxins impact different body systems and affect health. In the previous chapters, we looked at the statistics for chronic disease and mental health problems across the US.

Even if we think we are eating healthy, the quality of our food now is diminished, compared to what our grandparents were eating years ago. Dwindling mineral concentrations in fruits and vegetables was reported more than 15 years ago in England, by Professor Anne-Marie Mayer PhD. Donald Davis, biochemist at the University of Texas, has discovered, through his research, that over the last 50 years there has been significant decline in the protein, calcium, phosphorus, iron, riboflavin and vitamin C in conventionally grown fruits and vegetables. The protein in wheat has significantly diminished as well.

If we eat food that sends our bodies the wrong message, we set ourselves up for being overweight, under nourished, with possibility of heart disease, type 2 diabetes, arthritis and fatty liver disease.

Another illness that I truly believe is linked to the poor quality of food and environmental toxins is Metabolic Syndrome. National Heart Lung and Blood Institute defines it as: "group of symptoms that raises your risk of stroke, heart disease and type 2 diabetes". It is predicted that metabolic syndrome will overtake smoking as leading cause for heart disease. Risk factors include: large waistline; high triglyceride level; low HDL cholesterol level; high blood pressure; high fasting blood sugar. The National Institute says you need to have 3 of these factors to be diagnosed with Metabolic Syndrome. Along with the above risk factors, The Right Diagnosis lists other possible symptoms such as: depression; heart palpitations; fatigue; sleep apnea; memory problems. PLEASE, see your health care provider if you have any concerns about any health issues.

CHEMICALY SENSITIVE PERSONS

Miller (2001) observes that there is a unique pattern of illness involving chemically exposed groups worldwide, with multi-symptoms and new chemical, food, and drug intolerances. The one thing found in common is an initial chemical exposure event.

Exposure to neurotoxins can manifest in any of the following ways: irritability; depression; anxiety; paranoia; and psychosis. Milder neurotoxicity is seen with a range of toxins including: solvents; metals; and pesticides at currently permissible levels. Often syndromes are poorly defined and, in some cases, overlapping, including: Multiple Chemical Sensitivity; closed or sick building syndrome; Gulf War Syndrome; or Chronic Fatigue Syndrome. Lundberg (2001)

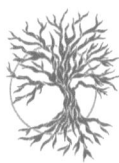

In a 9-year follow-up study with 18 chemically sensitive individuals, 15 met DSM-IV criteria for a mood disorder; 10 for an anxiety disorder. Self -report data showed little change over the course of 9 years. The 10 most frequent complaints attributed to chemical sensitivity were headache, memory loss, forgetfulness, sore throat, joint aches, trouble thinking, shortness of breath, back pain, muscle aches, and nausea (Black, 2001).

In my case, it was the incident of a faulty ventilation system in the office I worked, plus subsequent exposure to perfumes and cleaning chemicals. That was the tipping point (or tilting point) in my health. It started when one day I woke up with red, swollen eye lids, confusion and headaches. Later, came irritability, anxiety and panic, and finally depression. I was sent first to Occupational Health and later an allergist who found "nothing wrong with me". I was treated as if it were all in my head. Further, if I wanted an offending substance removed, I needed to present proof with the Material Safety Data Sheets that the substance was dangerous. If my symptoms didn't appear on the Material Safety Data Sheet, then that wasn't considered to be the offending substance, no matter what my experience was. I later became aware that companies do not have to list every ingredient or potential hazard in a product on the MSDS. Fragrance was not considered part of the problem, and elimination of fragrance in the office was denied as it was a person's 'right' to wear or have a fragrance in the office. I was also disbelieved, as they would say; "if it's such a problem with you, why aren't you sneezing?"

I'm sure you have heard the saying: It's the straw that broke the camel's back. Remember the phrase "body burden"? How it's not one chemical per se, but the total chemical load we are now exposed to in this society? Why is it that some people seem to go about life unscathed? Yet, for some, they get sick after one incident of toxic exposure, or, it happens more subtly - people just begin to notice that they are "just feeling crappy"; suffering from various chronic health issues in addition to emotional symptoms of depression, anxiety, confusion etc.? In other words, some people can no longer tolerate certain chemicals or exposures that never seemed to bother them prior.

Miller explains a possible new theory of disease, "Toxicant-Induced Loss of Tolerance" or ("TILT"). Miller believes that TILT has the potential to explain certain cases of asthma, migraine headaches, and depression, as well as chronic fatigue, fibromyalgia, and "Gulf War Syndrome."
Toxicant-Induced Loss of Tolerance is characterized by a profound breakdown in prior, natural tolerance, resulting from either acute or chronic exposure to chemicals (pesticides, solvents, indoor air contaminants, etc.), followed by (2) triggering of symptoms by small quantities of previously tolerated chemicals (traffic exhaust, fragrances, gasoline), foods, drugs, and food/drug combinations (alcohol, caffeine) (Miller C., 2001). It's a process of getting sick when

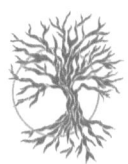

exposed to toxins, and then not being able to get better; often being retriggered upon smaller exposures in the future. Miller has also found that TILT emerges from more sensitive limbic systems.

When the term environment is used, most practitioners think of a person's family and immediate social circle. The physical environment is an important consideration as well. Anecdotal evidence indicates that clinicians see more and more patients who have been exposed to environmental poisons or stress. Much psychological suffering and disability is not due to major mental illness but to psychological or physical stress and trauma (Lundberg, 1998).

In the Annals of Family Medicine, July 2012, Miller et al, published a study of 400 primary care patients with chronic health issues, finding that 20 % (1 in 5) suffer from some degree of chemical intolerance. (Niemark,2013)

Regrettably, as debilitating as chemical sensitivity can be, it is not recognized by the World Health Organization or the American Medical Association. MCS is often associated with having a mental health condition as somatoform disorder, depression, or anxiety. As Dr. Anne Steinemann and Professor Stan Caress have discovered in their national epidemiological studies, chemical exposure will affect the brain in some way, however, chemical sensitivity is not caused by depression or anxiety.

WHAT IS THE ANSWER

If a disease is primarily related to exposure to toxic substances, one needs to avoid the exposure. The first step in environmental medicine is not a drug, not surgery, not a psychiatrist, but rather avoiding exposure. If doctors ignore the importance of nontoxic and non-allergenic environments, and return the injured person to chemically contaminated workplace while covering up their symptoms with medications, they are doing no one a favor. They have simply failed to address the source of the problem. (Ranheim, 2008).

In the field of environmental medicine, their understanding of toxicology has now accepted that there is no risk-free exposure, and that each individual responds differently. Dr. Claudia Miller recognizes that there is a "new pattern of illness and the strong relationship of chronic health problems—ranging from asthma and autoimmune disorders to ADHD and mood disorders—to common environmental exposures." (Miller, September 2008).

Dr. Claudia Miller has developed a validated questionnaire for assessing chemical intolerance called the QEESI (Quick Environmental Exposure and Sensitivity Inventory). It is to be used to identify patients with chemical sensitivities. This form is available at

http://drclaudiamiller.com/wp-content/uploads/2012/01/qeesi.pdf

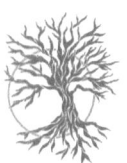

CHAPTER 8

Breaking Down the Bad Guys

This chapter contains information related to some of the main toxins and chemicals; this by no means is an exhaustive list. It is included so that you can have an awareness of these common toxins, where they are found and how they impact the body. Often, we hear something is an "endocrine disrupter" or a "neurotoxin" but what does that mean? Basically, this information is here to help increase your environmental vocabulary, which was very difficult for me in the beginning, and still is somewhat, to keep track of it all. Please refer to Appendix A – C in the end of this book.

NEUROTOXINS

Neurotoxins, a substance that is poisonous or destructive to nerve tissues, is found in metals, (especially Mercury, Manganese and Lead), pesticides, solvents, food additives, preservatives, and cosmetics.

In 1978, Tilson and Cabe reported on the adverse consequences people experienced because of exposure to neurotoxins. Symptoms were experienced in the sensory, motor, affective and associative areas, and are described as follows:

Sensory area included: loss of smell; a sensation of tingling or pricking "pins and needles" in the feet, fingers, and toes; visual deficits; extreme sensitivity to light; involuntary eye movement; reduced or limited vision; hearing deficits; tinnitus; perceptual dysfunctions and pseudo-hallucinations.

Motor areas were affected by symptoms such as: weakness in hands, arms, legs: paralysis, incoordination (inability to control voluntary muscular movements); dizziness; fatigue; tremor; convulsions; hyperactivity; and slurred speech.

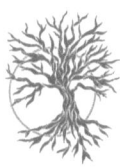

Affective (emotional) areas were affected by: nervousness; irritability; agitation; euphoria; psychosis; apathy; lethargy; depression; compulsive behavior.

Associative or cognitive symptoms were reported as impaired short term memory, impaired long term memory, confusion, and disorientation. Physiological responses included: disrupted sleep wake cycles; hypothermia; hyperthermia; sweating; loss of appetite; loss or gain in body weight (Tilson & Cabe, 1978).

PESTICIDES

Pesticides are often misunderstood to mean insecticides only. However, according to the EPA, the term Pesticide refers to any substance or mixture of substances intended for preventing, destroying, repelling or mitigating any pest. The term also applies to Herbicides (weed killers), fungicides, and various other substances used to control "pests"

In other words, Pesticides kill or repel "pests"- from the four-legged furry rodent variety to bugs, weeds and molds. They have been around since the 1940s. Consider the mosquito, and if you're in new England, instead of spring, we have black fly season. We often reach for sprays because we want them to kill those harmful pesky insects, but the ingredients in these insecticides are also toxic to humans, pets, birds, beneficial bugs, and the environment.

Human exposure may result in both acute and delayed health effects. Pesticide poisoning accounts for a significant number of deaths worldwide. In developing countries, the estimated annual death rate in agricultural workers is 18.2 per 100 000 full-time workers and 7.4 per million schoolchildren.

Delayed health effects associated with pesticide exposure include: leukemia; lymphomas; soft-tissue sarcomas; and brain, bone, and stomach cancers in farmers, sprayers, and production workers. A relationship between parental exposure and childhood cancers has been reported in human

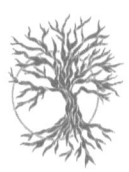

studies. Pesticides may play a role in the occurrence of Parkinson's disease and developmental defects (Bolognesi & F.D., 2011).

Side effects from pesticide exposure range from "mild symptoms of dizziness and nausea to serious, long-term neurological, developmental and reproductive disorders." Children are at greater risk because their organs are still developing and because they eat more, relative to their body weight (EPA, 2002).

There is a treasure trove of information on pesticides at Beyond Pesticides.org. I encourage you to check it out for yourselves. You can frankly spend hours there. "Beyond Pesticides" launched the Pesticide Induced Disease Databank, which enables access to epidemiologic and laboratory studies based on real world exposure that links public health effects to pesticides.

(Owens et al, 2010) reports that 19 of the 30 commonly used lawn pesticides are linked to cancer. Numerous studies also link pesticide exposure to: Asthma; Birth and Fetal defects; Cancers (Brain Cancer; Breast Cancer; Leukemia; Lymphoma; Prostate Cancer; and other); developmental and learning disorders; ADHD; Autism; Alzheimer's and Parkinson's; Diabetes (especially type 2). They are known to affect the endocrine system, which helps guide developmental growth, reproduction and behavior.

Researchers at Mt. Sinai School of Medicine, University of California Berkeley's School of Public Health, and Columbia University's Mailman School of Public Health, published three separate studies in April of 2011, showing a connection between prenatal exposure to organophosphate pesticides and diminished IQs in children between the ages of 6 and 9. (Release, 2011).

The National Institutes of Health study found:

> children with higher levels of organophosphate pesticides in their urine were much more likely to have attention deficit/hyperactivity disorder. (Bouchard, Bellinger, Wright, & Weisskoph, 2010).

Scientists fed 23 children conventionally - produced food for three days and then an all-organic diet for five days. Following the switch, pesticide metabolites in the children's urine decreased dramatically, demonstrating that:

> changing to an organic diet does in fact significantly decrease pesticide exposure.

This was the first study to use dietary intervention to assess children's exposure to pesticides. It provides new and persuasive evidence of the effectiveness of this intervention. (Lu, Toepel, Irish, Barr, & Bravo, 2006)

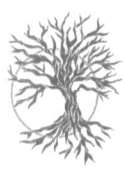

GLYPHOSATE

Chemical Watch Factsheet published by Beyond Pesticides has some great information about Glyphosate aka Roundup:

We see this product in stores everywhere. It is a registered herbicide with the EPA since 1974, increasing in popularity over the years, due to its claims of low toxicity and the promotion of GM crops engineered to be tolerant to Glyphosate.

Studies have reported that people exposed to Glyphosate are 2.7 times more likely to contract non-Hodgkin lymphoma. Agricultural Health Study found that Glyphosate had a suggested association with multiple myeloma. Glyphosate and its formulated products adversely affect embryonic, placental and umbilical cord cells, and impacts fetal development. Pre-pregnancy exposures to Glyphosate were found to moderately increase the risk for spontaneous abortions in mothers exposed to Glyphosate products.

Glyphosate is also linked to genetic damage and endocrine disruption, as well as environmental damage and water contamination. It is one of the most widely used and well known herbicides in the world.

A recent study published by Dr. Michael Antoniou and Dr. Robin Mesnage of Kings College in London, has linked Glyphosate to non-alcoholic fatty liver disease. Found primarily in over- weight and obese people, symptoms often include: fatigue, nausea, jaundice, cirrhosis, and abdominal pain. (Martin, K 2017) Other symptoms may include inability to lose weight, excess weight in the abdominal area, elevated cholesterol/triglyceride levels, indigestion, discomfort over the liver area. (RM Healthy)

GMO FOODS

Genetically modified organisms (GMOs) are living organisms whose genetic material, DNA, has been artificially manipulated, spliced, rearranged or eliminated through genetic engineering, not occurring in nature or through traditional crossbreeding or selective methods.

Almost all GMOs are "Roundup-Ready"- meaning they are made to withstand direct application of herbicide and/or produce an insecticide. Contrary to industry promises, the GMO traits have not resulted in increased yields, drought intolerance, enhanced nutrition, or any other benefit.

GMO safety has been a hotly contested issue in this country, although many other nations do not consider them safe. Australia, Japan, and the entire European Union restrict or ban production or sale of GMOs.

There is a growing body of evidence that connects GMOs with health problems, environmental damage, and violation of farmers' and consumer rights. Please see LIVING NON GMO, NON GMO Project's website for more.

In researching the health risks of GMO foods, I discovered CARE2 Health Living website. Their article on

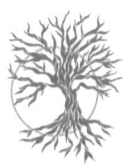

GMOs and The Four Potential Health risks of GMO foods is summarized below:

Unfortunately, if you are living in the US, you may have been eating GMO foods for years. Much of the field corn and soybeans produced (ones fed to livestock or used to provide fillers in processed foods), contain some portion of GMO material. It is also found in sugar produced from sugar beets and vegetable oils.

GMOs are often found in cereal, crackers, baking mixes, veggie burgers and even dairy. GMOs have infiltrated our store shelves with minimal study on the long-term health effects. Environmental Working Group estimates that each American consumes about 190 pounds of GM foods each year.

HEALTH CONCERNS

ALLERGIES: Genetic engineering can increase the levels of naturally occurring allergens already present in a food, or insert allergenic properties into a food that did not previously contain them. It can also result in brand new allergens we've never known.

ANTIBIOTIC RESISTANCE: Overuse of antibiotics can potentially cause the development of antibiotic-resistant pathogens.

PESTICIDE EXPOSURE: Most of GM crops are engineered to contain a gene for pesticide resistance. Most are "Roundup Ready," meaning they can be sprayed with Monsanto's glyphosate herbicide Roundup without being harmed.

UNKNOWN: Foreign genetic material can cause other genetic material in a host to behave erratically. Genes can be suppressed or overexpressed. One consequence of overexpression, for example, can be cancer. Nutritional problems can also result from the transfer. GM crops have been linked to health problems as diverse as reproductive damage, cancer, Alzheimer's disease and diabetes. Concerned scientists have been outspoken about these risks

IMPORTANT DISTINCTION:

Although choosing NON-GMO is good, there is an important distinction which I recently discovered. I was shopping at a specialty food store in York Maine. I noticed that some products were labeled ORGANIC and some were only labeled NON-GMO. I stood there; Which to choose, which to choose, and does it matter?

YES!

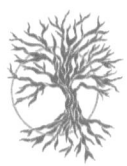

All food that has a label ORGANIC is also NON-GMO.

Only the ORGANIC label is certifies that there are NO pesticides; Roundup Herbicides; no sewer sludge (commonly known as bio-solids); no antibiotics, and humanely treated animals.

However, not all food with the NON-GMO label is organic. Non-GMO crops can be grown in the same manner as conventional crops.

Truth in Labeling: Organic certification can be a confusing and controversial subject. Some small business and small local farms say they cannot afford the certification process to allow them to be labeled as organic. So, **ask** them about their ingredients and methods before you write them off.

 To add more confusion to this issue, there are also 3 different levels of organic; "100 Percent Organic" which is the highest standard, then, "USDA organic", then last, "Made with Organic Ingredients" Check out the USDA's site on Organic Standards for more information.

https://www.ams.usda.gov/grades-standards/organic-standards

PETROCHEMICALS

Petrochemicals are found in our everyday products. They are made from crude oil and natural gas. In 1859, C. Edwin Drake struck oil, and the US petroleum industry was born. According to the American Petroleum Institute, this industry adds aproximately $1 trillion dollars to the US economy and provides and suports over 9 million american jobs. Petrochemicals have been around since WWI.

The American Fuel and Petrochemical Manufacturers trade association lists some very useful and important products, which I will break down on the following page. There are some things I am sure you will be surprised and perhaps a bit frightened to find out. One thing for sure, petrochemicals are everywhere. However, I don't want them on my body or in my food. We need to find ways to reduce our exposure as much as possible.

Petrochemicals are classified in three catagories based on chemical structure.

1. Olefins: the industrial chemicals – plastic products; synthetic rubber; propylene; butadiene and ethylene.

    PROPYLENE: adhesives; appliances; battery cases and parts; carpeting; coatings; cups; containers; caps/closures; crates; diapers; fixtures;

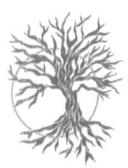

PROPYLENE (cont:) housewares; film and sheet packaging; fibers and filaments; furniture; insulation; laminates; paints.

BUTADIENE: automotive bumper bars; automotive trim components; keyboard keys; golf club heads; tires; hoses and belts; latex paints; kitchen appliances; rubber; toys.

ETHYLENE: artificial joints; bags; bearings; clothing; credit cards; detergent bottles; electrical cables; engine coolant; film; gears; milk jugs; pipes; polyester; siding; signs; tubing; IV/blood bags.

2. Aromatics – dyes , synthetic detergents, plastics and synthetic fiber. Benzeine, Toluene and xylene.

BENZENE: automotive headlamps; cutlery; computer cases; instrument stings; nylons; phones; packaging material; petri dishes; rope; safety glasses; sunglasses; tents; test tubes.

XYLENE: automotive applications; beverage bottles; carpets; fabrics; electronics; lumber; photographic film; solvents; sportswear textiles.

TOLUENE: bedding; boats; fabric; food casings; furniture; nylon textiles; clothing; upholstery; varnish.

3. Synthetic Gas. Mixture of carbon monoxide and hydrogen. Used to make amonia (fertilizer) and methanol (solvents)

Petrochemicals are also found in: **food; pharmaceuticals; health and beauty products; household products; household cleaners; cars; computers; cell phones; childrens toys; pesticides; fertilizers. Choosing organic products helps reduce your petrochemical exposure.**

Petrochemicals and their bi products, such as dioxin, are known to cause serious health problems.

> Although they are an important part of our lives, (depending on how they are used), they can also hazardous to our health and to the environment. Since these chemicals can be absored though the skin and injested, they can accumulate in the tissues and organs causing brain, nerve and liver damage, birth defects and cancer, asthma, hormonal disorders and allergies. (Shukla 2010)

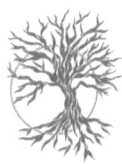

FOOD ADDITIVES AND PRESERVATIVES

In 2008, the Center for Science in the Public Interest (CSPI) in Washington DC petitioned the FDA to ban artificial food dyes because of their connection to behavioral problems in children.

> CSPI has concluded that there are nine artificial dyes used in the US that are carcinogenic and cause hypersensitivity reactions and behavior problems. (Potera, 2010).

Food additives and preservatives are chemicals added to our food. Artificial dyes are derived from petroleum and are found in thousands of foods and other products. For thirty years, there has been evidence linking artificial food dyes to behavioral problems in children. Adults are also affected. Some of the immediate effects may cause headaches or alter your energy level, or they may affect your mental concentration, behavior, or immune response. Those with long-term effects could increase your risk of cancer, cardiovascular disease and other degenerative conditions.

A further description of twelve common additives and their effects on health is found in Appendix B.

The FDA does not require manufacturers to test dyes for developmental neurotoxicity. In Europe, as of July 2010, most foods that contain artificial dyes must carry labels warning they may cause hyperactivity in children. (Barrett, 2007; Haas 1996; Weiss, 2000).

There are indeed enduring controversies over the use of contemporary and alternative medicine (CAM) for the treatment of ADHD. CAM supports elimination of artificial food additives, colors, preservatives and sugar, as well as yoga and bio feedback. More rigorously designed studies are needed to evaluate their effectiveness as a single therapy for ADHD. (Rojas, 2005)

MONOSODUIM GLUTAMATE

MSG is a popular preservative and is found in many food items. When considering if a product has MSG or not, labels are often misleading and confusing. If a label on a product states that there is no MSG, one would think they were safe. However, there are over forty food ingredients besides "monosodium glutamate" (MSG) that contain MSG or create MSG during the ingredient's production.

Because of FDA regulations, they are called by their common name such as "autolyzed yeast," "maltodextrin," "sodium caseinate," and "soy sauce". They are so common that the consumer has no clue that there is MSG in the ingredient. (Truth In Labeling).

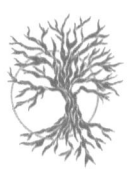

The FDA admits that "short term reactions" known as MSG Symptom complex, effects certain groups of people. These symptoms include: numbness, burning, tingling, facial pressure or tightness, chest pain, difficulty breathing, nausea, rapid heartbeat, dizziness and weakness. (Mercola)

ARTIFICIAL SWEETNERS

Sweeteners have grown in popularity with individuals wanting to cut out sugar. Aspartame has been the most controversial. Dr. Ralph Walton compiled a list of ninety studies conducted on humans and animals, and found eighty-three of them found one or more problems related to Aspartame. Seventy-four studies conducted by the Aspartame industry claimed no problems were found (Walton, 1993).

Aspartame, aka known as NutraSweet (often in sugar free or diet products), is found in over six thousand products ranging from foods, beverages, laxatives, vitamins and pharmaceuticals. Reports have linked the use of aspartame to birth defects, cancer, diabetes, epilepsy, seizures and emotional disorders. (Mercola)

FRAGRANCE

It was not until I tried to eliminate fragrance from my life that I realized how fragrance infiltrates everything in our lives. Fragrance is in most everything from personal care products, household products, air fresheners, and children's products. Fragrance is also used in food, beverages and flavorings.

The International Fragrance Association, due to consumer pressure finally published a list of chemicals that its members use in their products. 3,163 chemicals were reported. An analysis of these chemicals showed cause for concern. Many are highly hazardous and contain hormone disrupters. (Frack, Sutton, 2010).

There are not only health concerns but environmental concerns, as fragrances are volatile organic compounds (VOCs) as well, which add to indoor and outdoor air pollution. Synthetic musk compounds are persistent in the environment and contaminate water and aquatic life. There is little governmental regulation of fragrance (Bridges, 2002).

Fragrance chemicals and synthetic musks are also turning up in human breast milk. Synthetic musks are used to mask chemical odors in products labeled "unscented." Kannan, an environmental toxicologist at the New York State Department of Health, studied milk samples collected from 39 nursing women in Massachusetts, and found the highest levels of musks ever recorded in nursing mothers. The average concentration was five times higher than that of European breast milk samples 10 years ago.

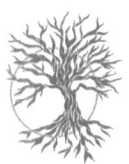

Musk ingredients often are not listed on product labels, or they are called simply "fragrance" or by the trade names galaxolide (for HHCB) or onalide (for AHTN) (Potera, 2005).

Health concerns related to fragrance are found to impact the skin, respiratory, and neurological areas. Olfactory pathways are the most direct connection to the brain of any of our senses and provide a means of toxin materials entering the brain. Fragrance has been cited as a trigger for conditions such as asthma, allergies and migraine headaches.

Dr. Steinemann's research has confirmed that there is a prevalence of fragrance sensitivity among individuals, and fragrance products can trigger adverse health effects. (34.7 % of the population report health problems such as migraines and respiratory difficulties, 15.1 % have lost workdays or a job due to fragrance exposure in the workplace). Because fragrances are so prevalent, it's almost impossible to avoid them, especially in public. 20.2 % would enter a business and then leave as quick as possible if they smelled air fresheners or some fragrance product. Over half the population surveyed would prefer fragrance - free workplaces and health care facilities. (Steinemann 2016).

Individuals with Multiple Chemical Sensitivity or environmental illness are especially vulnerable, as fragrance has often contributed to the illness onset or exacerbated an already existing condition. The individual fragrance ingredients have been associated with neurotoxicity, cancer and other adverse health effects. (Suzuki)

Dr. Steinemann investigated what some of these chemicals where and what limits their disclosure. She found that after analyzing six best-selling air fresheners and laundry products, nearly 100 VOCs were identified, none of the VOCs were listed on any product label, and one was listed on one material safety data sheets (MSDS). Ten of the identified VOCs are regulated as toxic or hazardous under federal laws, with three (acetaldehyde, chloromethane, and 1,4-dioxane) classified as Hazardous Air Pollutants (HAPs). She also found that these ingredients are not listed on product labels, as no law in the U.S. requires disclosure of all chemical ingredients in consumer products or in fragrances. (Steinemann, 2008) .

In a 2015 study, Steinemann found that fragranced products emit a range of VOCs, but few are disclosed to the public. She found that more than 156 VOCs were emitted from 37 fragranced consumer products. Of these 156 VOCs, 42 were classified as toxic or hazardous under US Federal Law. Importantly, emissions of carcinogenic hazardous air pollutants from so called "green or organic fragranced products were not significantly different from regular fragranced products.

Unfortunately, even products making a claim of being "green" (such as "organic," "natural," with "essential oils" or "organic perfume"), emitted just as many toxic and hazardous compounds and probable carcinogens as the

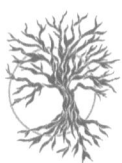

standard products. Half of the products emitted one or more carcinogenic "hazardous air pollutants" (1,4-dioxane, acetaldehyde, formaldehyde, and methylene chloride), which have no safe exposure level, according to the U.S. Environmental Protection Agency. Steinman further explains that even if a product doesn't contain hazardous chemicals, it can generate them. For instance, limonene, which was the most common chemical emitted from these products, reacts with ozone in surrounding air to create a range of potentially hazardous secondary pollutants, such as formaldehyde, acetaldehyde (Steineman, 2010).

We may think we are safe if we do not smell anything, but studies in Sweden found that the lowest concentration level in which a chemical causes irritant effects might be below odor threshold level. Studies of brain waves suggest that chemicals present in ambient air may affect the nervous system without our being conscious of it. (Nimmermark, 2004).

Fragrance is also used to cover up the odor of other materials in a product and does not have to be listed as fragrance in the ingredients. Masking fragrance is often used in 'unscented" and 'fragrance free' products. Any material may be used as a fragrance ingredient and most often is petrochemical in nature. The individual components do not have to be listed on the label, The fragrance portion alone may contain over 100 chemicals. Trade secrecy is often required to protect the formulas. (Steinemann, 2008)

PHTHALATES

Phthalates are esters of phthalic acid and are mainly used to make fragrance products last longer, make plastics flexible, and act as lubricants in cosmetics. They are also in additives to hairsprays, wood finishers and lubricants. Phthalates are widely known as endocrine disrupters – hormone disrupters.

Phthalate exposure has been linked to early puberty in girls, reduced sperm count in men, birth defects in the developing male fetus, obesity and insulin resistance in men, and Health Canada notes that exposure may cause liver or kidney failure in young children when products are sucked or chewed for extended periods.

Stay away from fragrances/perfume, and if you must have a scent, choose organic essential oils. Beware! Natural Vanilla Fragrance does not mean "safe". It means chemicals were used to produce the vanilla smell! Eliminate plastic whenever possible, eat organic produce, meat or dairy, because phthalates are used in pesticides or conventional agriculture.

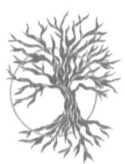

CHAPTER 9
FINAL THOUGHTS

To adopt the stance that environmental toxins are the sole cause for every single medical or emotional symptom would be irresponsible. What I am saying is that there needs to be a holistic approach by looking at presenting symptoms along with lifestyle and exposures to toxins. In her book, Anxiety: Hidden Causes, Sharon Heller, PhD quotes the following statistics, found in recent studies, that there are over fifty medical conditions that can cause prominent anxiety symptoms.

In one psychiatric facility, forty-six percent of patients suffered medical problems that caused or contributed to their anxiety. Finally, Joan Rittenhouse, of the National Institute of Mental Health, concluded that up to eighty one percent of all psychiatric patients probably have misdiagnosed physical disorders, including potentially lethal misdiagnosed cancers. (Heller, 2010).

Considering these statistics, is it any wonder that the seven individuals of my study could not find an answer for their problems? One source of frustration were people were being discounted or not getting help from their providers. In some cases, the treatment was worse than the symptoms. If the lens of environmental illness were added as an extra assessment tool, perhaps these people would find help sooner.

A simple screening tool, such as Miller's QEESI, or adding questions to the intake process to inquire what products a person uses would be a good place to start. Current health questionnaires often capture symptoms such as headaches, sleep patterns, anxiety, and other related issues. A section giving a glimpse to the exposure an individual has to certain toxins would be a good place to begin. Which cleaning and personal care products do you use? What does your daily diet consist of?

For example, Johnny's mom is bringing him in for counseling because he is angry, aggravated, has headaches, stomach pains and can't sleep. With this lifestyle assessment,

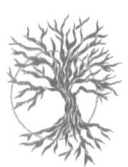

if you discover that he spends a lot of time in front of the computer eating nothing but processed foods, such as Slim Jims, Doritos, Hot Pockets, Ramen Noodles, Mountain Dew and Red Bull during the course of the week, chances are some simple modifications in his diet and routine may help. Also, therapy will not be beneficial if some of the symptoms are caused by toxins in the diet.

I believe that it is the responsibility of mental health centers, medical practices, clinics, hospitals and schools to be healthy environments that are free of toxins and fragrances. These places should also provide educational materials to consumers regarding the latest research and information related to toxins and what people can do to avoid them. It should be clear, concise and with easy to understand product alternatives. People are more apt to make healthy choices if the information is readily available. People in this study were overwhelmed by the process because of the lack of good information.

Physicians for Social Responsibility is one organization that provides information and training materials to consumers, as well as health practitioners, regarding the dangers of some environmental toxins. That is a good place to start, but we can do more. We need to bridge the gap between the professions and adopt a more holistic approach. Share the knowledge. This topic needs to be more widely accepted and practiced in the health community, as well as schools and other institutions.

I come away with more questions because of this study. Is the motivating factor for wellness related to a person's belief that they have control over situations and events in their lives? Do people who take an active role in their health tend to be healthier? The knowledge of the effects of various toxic exposures is available, yet how do we begin to build the bridge between all the individuals involved? How do health professionals provide better care?

Further recommendations come from the advocacy standpoint. Insurance coverage is a major factor in people not getting help sooner. Environmental Medicine, as well as many other contemporary and alternative medicines, are not covered by insurance, so people do not experience the benefits and knowledge that these approaches could offer. If CAM were offered under the umbrella of traditional care, then perhaps insurance would cover it. Considering toxic exposures within traditional practice would bridge this gap until the day when insurance covers alternative medicine.

Finally, there is a societal myth that governmental organizations and corporations protect the consumer. The fact was clear in the literature review that governmental agencies do little to protect consumers, and, there is more misinformation on labels than truth. A product is deemed safe until proven unsafe. Many consumers do not know this. "I thought that if it was on the shelf it was safe" or "they wouldn't sell it if it wasn't good for you." Education is the key.

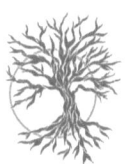

CHAPTER 10

SOLUTIONS

If you've made it to this point in the book, Congratulations! You did it! I think it takes a lot of courage and resolve to absorb all this information.

Maybe you are inspired and excited to get going on a healthy new path. Wonderful!

Or, maybe by now you might feel a bit overwhelmed. Maybe you think "I can't even go there, it's too much, so I won't even try!"   Maybe you're in a bit of a panic, thinking everything around you is poison, and you don't know where to begin. It feels like Mt. Everest.

Maybe you're thinking: "Yah, nope! Not for me!"

Believe me, its ok. I've been there before.

In this chapter, I present a plan to follow if you want to begin to make some changes. I'm not putting this out there as the "be all, end all" expert plan, but these are simply suggestions based on my own research and life experience.

To those who think this isn't for you, maybe consider trying some of these suggestions for a couple of months, just to see if there is any difference in the way you feel.

Remember: Change can be hard, even if it's a positive thing! Remember: Don't panic. Breathe.

The good news is that we have come a long way in the eight years since I started my journey to a healthy lifestyle. There are so many great resources and websites now with good and accurate information.

I can help you with a plan so as not to get totally overwhelmed.

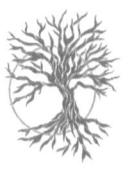

FIRST STEP

Focus on what you want to create now, moving forward.

Focus on healthy living and making mindful healthy choices!

Keep Fear Out of the Process!

It's important for you to know that the changes I made came in stages. It didn't happen all at once. It takes time. Frankly, I didn't have all the informational resources available to me then, as there is now, so a lot of the process was difficult. I didn't have the money to throw everything out and start fresh, either. Eliminating products and replacing them with healthier alternatives was a slow process - especially eliminating fragrance products. I learned quickly that shopping in the grocery store aisle was a waste of time. I also discovered, when simply shopping in the organic stores for organic health and beauty products, that some of those harmful ingredients were still on the labels. Fragrance was often one of them.

Because fragrance was such a prominent health issue for my partner, I eliminated that first. Soon after that, elimination of toxins in cleaners became a priority due to my own chemical injury. At that time, I wasn't even tackling the food issue, although I didn't eat at fast food restaurants. At that time, I wasn't concerned with organic or non-organic. I needed to get control of one topic at a time. Feel free to choose where you would like to start.

THE BODY

PERSONAL CARE PRODUCTS

Think of all the products you use for personal care. Take a walk into your bathroom and see all the soaps, shampoos, conditioners, lotions, deodorant, toothpaste, shaving cream, after shave, lotions, potions, beauty products cologne, perfume etc. Men and women have their own separate stuff, and even kids and babies do as well.

I'm quite sure you have a lot of money invested in these products. And it may feel a bit unnerving to just toss hundreds of dollars' worth in the trash.

The choice of how you proceed is up to you.

PERFUMES-FRAGRANCE

Eliminate entirely! With the number of chemicals present, I'm not seeing this as a healthy risk. I avoid fragrance entirely. Fragrance, as you remember, is prevalent. Look on the label of your products. If it contains the word perfume, parfum, or fragrance, it is full of chemicals. Even "unscented" or "fragrance free" may contain masking chemicals.

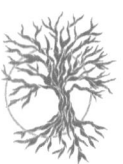

SOAP

I eliminated all body washes, moisturizing soaps and deodorant soaps, and I replaced those with Kirks castile soap then on to Dr. Bonners. I later discovered that Dr. Bonners is truly a "magic soap" that you can use in many ways! My personal favorite was 18-in-1 Hemp Unscented Baby Mild Pure Castile Soap, made with organic oils. That is a staple in my home. I have since taken to soap making as a hobby, and I now make my own fragrance - free organic castile soap – which is a wonderful combination of organic olive oil and coconut oil. My husband uses it to shave, eliminating the need for shaving cream! By the way, I don't own stock or get kickbacks from advertising my favorite products!

SHAMPOO & HAIR CARE

I then tackled the fragrance-free issue with shampoos and conditioners. It was nearly impossible to find something fragrance - free in the health and beauty aisle at that time, so on to internet shopping I went. Again, even in organic stores, many of the products still contain fragrance and other chemicals. Also, beware of phthalates.

I simply do not waste my time in the health and beauty aisle (now that's an oxymoron) of grocery stores or drug stores. I typically shop for these products in organic sections or in the Natural Food stores. I am also cautious at natural stores, because some of the "natural" products contain fragrance, which is also loaded with, say it with me, chemicals. Some of the my early choices were Desert Essence and Stony Brook .

One of the things I discovered, which is common in most health and beauty products, is that certain ingredients often create a cycle of drying out the skin and hair, requiring us to then use lotions, potions and conditioners. I have since replaced the fragrance-free products with the Dr. Bronner's, 18-in1 Hemp Unscented Baby Mild Pure Castile Soap and, when I feel I need a conditioner, I use a bit of organic coconut oil.

HAIR COLOR

I also gave up coloring my hair, which I had been doing since my 20s. I discovered that most hair dyes have carcinogenic ingredients. There is also no such thing as organic hair dye, as most contain synthetic ingredients. The only "natural" hair color would be products like henna or other vegetables.
Before I just decided to give it up all together and embrace the grey, I went to less toxic products such as Herbatint and Naturtint.
NOTE: Since I switched to Dr. Bronner's and Coconut Oil, and stopped coloring my hair, I have the best feeling hair I have ever had in my entire life!

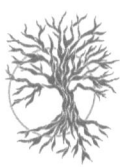

MOISTURIZERS

After getting rid of soaps that contained fragrances and other harmful ingredients, and using either my own homemade soap or the Dr. Bronner's, I discovered that my skin was not as dry! Nice trade off! I no longer needed to slather on moisturizer daily. When I do, I use the organic coconut oil. Which brings me to:

MAKEUP

A lot of the traditional beauty products do the same thing as creating a cycle of drying out the skin (through alcohols and such) and then we need to moisturize.

Remember: a lot of the traditional products contain petrochemicals and plasticizers and fragrances.

I remember thinking: Do I want to put crude oil on my skin? HECK NO!

At the time, I did not find any healthy alternative products for makeup, which I wore all the time. This included foundations, concealers, blush, eye shadow, mascara, and lipstick. Reluctantly, I went without and just used mascara.

I'm thinking of the phrase "harm reduction" here.

Sometimes it can get obsessive, so I try to remind myself that we are not striving for perfection. As I know better, I do better. Simple as that.

Later on, I found some less toxic options such as Mineral Fusion. This is still a really tough issue as most makeup products still contain some harmful ingredients.

According to Environmental Working Group (EWG) – Rejuva, (which I have not tried personally) and Mineral Fusion are top rated products. I could find no information on Bare Minerals. We could go on for pages about beauty products. The point is, no matter what the label claims, do your own research. EWGs Skin Deep resource is a great place to do your research.

DEODORANT

My key priority was to eliminate aluminum (linked to breast cancer) and fragrance. I now use Toms of Maine Unscented or the crystal. I am also in the process of making my own, which is always, in my opinion, the better option. It's a combination of equal parts ¼ c baking soda, 1/4 c organic cornstarch or arrowroot, and then mixing in enough organic coconut oil to make a paste, not to exceed 1/2 c. You can also add essential oils - 1/8 t to 1/4 t. Research the web for other recipes. If you're home on the weekend, out in the garden, feel free to go without! (you won't attract as many bugs!)

TOOTHPASTE

The fluoride issue can be controversial. I have switched to Toms fluoride free and no longer use mouthwash. I also use baking soda on occasion.

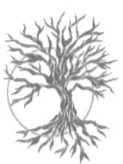

VITAMINS, SUPPLEMENTS, OTC DRUGS

What I found was most of them are made from the Big Pharma companies. This included a lot of what is considered over the counter health medicines. They are made from synthetically derived ingredients, artificial colors, flavors, petrochemicals, and GMO fillers. I have tried to eliminate as many Big Pharma products by looking to nature, using organic herbal teas and other natural remedies. There are some health care practitioners who are recommending natural supplements and vitamins to treat mild to moderate depression and anxiety in lieu of pharmaceuticals. My advice is: consumer, beware. Read the labels. Do your research. Consult with knowledgeable health practitioners. Just because it's from nature, does not mean it is harmless. **And – if you are on prescription medications – before you make any changes, Consult with your health care provider!**

BUG REPELLANT

Here, in New England, that can be a huge challenge. In black fly season, or what other parts of the country call spring, I use a combination of hair nets, long sleeves and avoid dark clothes, which attracts them. I go out before I shower. Just think about how common perfume products attract bugs! I burn citronella oil candles and apply peppermint oil as a deterrent. I also have planted mosquito repelling plants. I find those options are less toxic then DEET.

HOUSEHOLD

Start with the basics, where you live and breathe. Bottom line is that although there are a lot of alternative cleaning products on the market, with just three simple ingredients you can save a ton of money (who doesn't want to do that) and know that it is safe for you, your family and the environment. The three simple ingredients are:

Baking Soda, Vinegar and Water!

DEODORIZERS – SPRAYS – SCENTED CANDLES

The first thing I did was to get rid of all the deodorizers, sprays, plug - in air fresheners and scented candles. Believe me, with three teenage boys in the house, I had a lot. Remember anything labeled FRAGRANCE has hundreds of toxins and chemicals. Watch out for fragrance added to the trash bags now! Even if its "comforting lavender fragrance", and they advertise them as "mood" improvers, but get rid of all of them. That includes the ones hanging in your car, as well as and the plug-in versions. They are toxic.

Instead, choose unscented candles/tea lights. Not in your car of course! If you want a natural scent, try flowers!

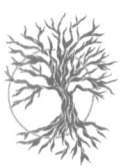

ODORS

To combat odors in the bathroom, this simple trick will do:

Light a match!

Let it burn for a few seconds, then simply blow it out and discard the stem in a small dish; empty when it's full. Having company over? Simply light a tea light or larger unscented candle in the bathroom. Remember: open those windows if you can.

Baking Soda is a very good product for eliminating unpleasant odors. Leave some in a dish or bowl under furniture, away from little hands or little paws; sprinkle a bit on the carpet, wait a bit, then vacuum; sprinkle some in shoes. There are numerous uses for baking soda!

CLEANING AND LAUNDRY

There are a lot of eco-friendly alternatives on the market now, but remember: stay away from petroleum – based products. Again, anything that says fragrance, albeit plant based, is still a chemical.

DISH AND LAUNDRY SOAPS

A few of my favorites are: Earth Friendly, ECOVER and Seventh Generation.   I am still working on perfecting homemade dish and laundry soap.

If you get rid of the petrochemical - based laundry products and switch to a more natural alternative, you will no longer need dryer sheets! Get rid of them! Common laundry products and dryer sheets leave a residue on your clothes, where scent and chemicals, linger.   When I began to eliminate these products, I noticed the heavy perfume scent on all my clothing (which was left over from all the traditional laundry products I had been using). I also tend to shop at thrift stores and noticed the same thing.   To eliminate fragrances (the molecules have burs on them to help them attach to things), I soaked them in distilled white vinegar for several hours prior to washing. That seems to eliminate the fragrance odor.

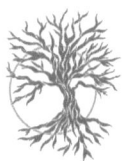

WINDOWS, COUNTERTOPS & OTHER CLEANUP

First, let me say that I understand that for certain areas of the home, we are interested in a near 100 % kill rate for germs. I get it. You don't have to use toxic chemicals to get that result. Is vinegar effective in killing germs? I don't want you to take just my word for it, as I have been using it, but according to the David Suzuki Foundation,

> "Yes. Acetic acid, or white vinegar, is a great disinfectant. It also acts as a deodorizer and cuts grease. And you can tackle household bacteria like salmonella, E. coli and other "gram-negative" bacteria with vinegar. Gram-negative bacteria can cause infections, including pneumonia, bloodstream infections, wound or surgical site infections, and meningitis. In fact, Heinz has unveiled a stronger version of its white distilled vinegar. Instead of five per cent acetic acid, it has six, which boosts the strength by 20 per cent. They're calling this new formula...wait for it..."cleaning" vinegar!

 For all other household cleaning, I purchased a glass spray bottle and mix 50 % distilled white vinegar and 50 % water. Sometimes I add a drop of tea tree oil as a disinfectant. I never use air fresheners. I have also wiped my cutting board with hydrogen peroxide and then rinsed with water.   I use baking soda and vinegar for my oven cleaner.

BATHROOM

I use baking soda, or borax, in combination with my vinegar water spray. If I have mildew or mold, which I seldom do, I use straight vinegar and let it set.

What's interesting to note is that soap scum is virtually eliminated since switching away from petrochemical-based soaps. Cleaning is a breeze. Seriously.

WINDOWS

Windows can also be cleaned with the vinegar and water mix. No more toxic window cleaner. No more wipes or harsh disinfectants. This mix does the trick.

Get rid of window cleaners, furniture polish, wipes, kitchen cleaners, bathroom cleaners. You will save a ton of money and space if you can keep the basics and make up your own. The Queen of Green has her own green cleaning recipes at: David Suzuki Foundation website. (Queen)

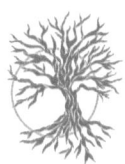

GENERAL HOUSEHOLD

Overall, I find it's about making smarter choices.   I am inevitably faced with new information daily about something or other that is now toxic. We can become fearful and obsessed, or we can simply make smarter healthier choices. I do the best I can, but sometimes we have to use products that contain some harmful ingredients.

Take paint for example. We recently remodeled our kitchen, and some of the adhesives, paints and varnishes-well those can be toxic! We try to choose the best brand, NO VOC etc., but frankly through experience we found some of the paint so far has been less than stellar in performance. What we do is to plan ahead. If we have to paint, then we do so in the time of the year that we can open up the house and let the off-gassing take place, and we leave the area for a bit. Also, be sure to wear masks.

Bags: Don't contribute to the plastic problem. Recycle or use cloth shopping bags or baskets. Seriously, I forget sometimes. I choose paper, when possible, because it can be recycled or used for mulch//weed cover in my yard.

You cannot eliminate toxins from your life, but you can make a choice not to have it on your body or in your food. Switch to healthier alternatives as they come to your awareness.

FOOD

This can be a hard one as we all have our favorite flavors, snacks and such, and often household budgets can be a factor. I also know that many people have no interest or time to cook from scratch, or grow their own food or raise their own chickens! Just start somewhere.

Water: Drink water. Eliminate the habit of using plastic bottled water. Plastic harms the environment and is not healthy for you. Plus, believe it or not, that hefty price you pay does not guarantee purity. If need be, invest in a water filter for your home.

The important thing is to eat whole foods. Eat more unrefined, unprocessed foods. Eat more whole grains. Eat things found in nature, rather than something that's in a cellophane package! Eat something that grow on trees or comes from the ground. Choose organic as much as possible. GMO foods often have limited taste or nutritional value. I discovered this when I was eating non-organic apples and pears. Their texture was so different. They often tasted like wet cardboard.

Your produce sticker should have a 5 digit PLU code beginning with a 9 for it to be organic.

Also, try to eat fruits and veggies in season. They will be fresher.

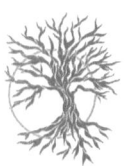

If you have kids, this can be tricky as you introduce new foods and eliminate unhealthy favorites. See if your favorites have organic alternatives. There is a wide variety of organic products now because along with specialty stores most supermarkets also have organic sections.

READ THE LABEL. Just because something says its organic, doesn't mean its "healthy". What I mean here is that your tasty snack may still have high calories, sugar, fat or carbs. So, you still shouldn't eat a whole box of cookies just because it says its organic! Also, canned soups may have a lot of sodium as opposed to making your own soup at home.

Also, beware that the term NATURAL and ORGANIC are not interchangeable; you may also see "all natural" "free range" "hormone free". Some companies use these terms as a marketing ploy, to make you think you're heating healthy. "All natural" can still contain chemicals, additives and preservatives". If you want to be sure its organic, then look for the word "organic".

Eliminate additives/preservatives and synthetic colors and dyes. **Appendix B is a guide of what to avoid for additives and preservatives.**

Perhaps a good place to start, instead of feeling like you must throw everything away in your cupboards, (which when I started this process, I certainly couldn't afford to do) is that each time you run out of something and have to replace it, replace it with an organic version.

That's how I got started. As things ran out and needed to be replaced, and each time I went shopping, I chose an organic version. I replaced the foods I used the most. Try switching out some of your daily products to organic ones- coffee for example, or cereal, or staple products: ketchups, spreads, salad dressings, etc.

I understand that going totally organic can be a bit expensive, especially when it comes to replacing your proteins (meat and chicken, etc.). I have found that, overall, produce is not that much more expensive - especially when you buy things that are in season. Think of the long-term health benefits.

Since I now have a yard and the time, I have also started a garden, and I grow from NON-Monsanto, non-GMO organic seeds and plants. I had to do lots of research on finding healthy seeds.

Environmental Working Group has the "clean 15 and dirty dozen" list, which is great for helping you replace fruits and vegetables, if you need to decide which ones are most necessary to have organic (if you can't do totally organic). I included it in **APPENDIX C** in the back of the book. There is a more comprehensive list on their website. EWG and has a good research area for foods.

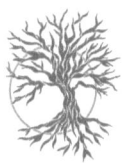

Along with that list, I would also add the following for important organic replacements:

Potatoes: (USDA found over 81% of potatoes in 2006 contained pesticides, even after washing and peeling).

Proteins: Beef, chicken, etc.; (think of all the hormones and anti-biotics often injected). Conventional deli meat is also full of additives and preservatives.

Milk, Dairy: Conventionally raised cows are given rBGH hormones, which is banned in other countries, and the American Cancer society acknowledges potential harm.

Apples, strawberries, kale and spinach: USDA study found over 58 pesticide residues in spinach!

I am not even going to delve into food intolerances, gluten free, vegetarian or vegan diets.   That's not what this book is about. Feel free to do your own research in this area. As for me, I'm working towards going gluten free now, and I can say that it has been a major factor in improved health since I have done so!

CONCLUSION

I think we can agree that chemicals do have their place in modern society. I also realize that I cannot eliminate everything harmful from my life 100 percent.

Harm Reduction is the key.
Intentional, wise, healthy, and informed choices,
are in your control.

What is important is to realize that it's the TOXIC LOAD we endure - the daily combinations and exposure to toxins - -as some of these chemicals are so pervasive. Sure, I need petrochemicals to run my car, type on this computer, or use my cell phone. However, I do NOT need them in my food or in my body. This is where we have the opportunity to make healthy choices.

Eliminating exposure to toxins, whenever possible for children, is crucial! Their tiny little bodies metabolize things at a much different rate than adults. Their developing brain is also at risk. This should be key for children of all ages and stages. Give them a healthy start! I wish I had this knowledge when I was raising mine!

I hope this book has given you some information to consider, along with help on where to begin your journey of health and wellbeing. God Bless!

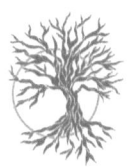

Appendix A
Summary of Chemicals EWG's Study
Chemicals found in Umbilical Cord Blood

BPA - is a petrochemical derivative used to toughen polycarbonate plastic and epoxy resin. It is found in food, beverages and packaging. The health risks of BPA are that it acts as a synthetic estrogen that disrupts the endocrine system and causes other harmful effects, even at very low doses.

Perchlorate - is a rocket fuel oxidizer that powers missiles, the space shuttle, fireworks, road flares, automobile airbags and more. The FDA detected perchlorate in 74 percent of 285 popular foods and beverages tested, including baby food. The health risks are that it can block the formation of thyroid hormones critical to brain development and growth in the fetus, infants, and children. Inadequate iodine intake increases the risk of perchlorate- related compromise of thyroid hormone production.

Perfluorochemicals (PFCs) - Teflon and Scotchguard chemicals PFCs are stain- and grease-proofing chemicals used in a variety of consumer products, such as carpets and furniture, as stain and grease repellents, in Teflon cookware, food packaging and clothing. PFCs have also been found in drinking water and certain food groups such as fruits and vegetables. PFCs are linked to a broad range of health risks, including decreased birth weight, reproductive problems, and elevated cholesterol.

Lead - is a neurotoxic metal that concentrates in the brain. It is found in lead paint and lead solder and brass plumbing fixtures in older homes. Although lead was banned in gasoline and paint decades ago, many other uses remain. It is still found in a variety of consumer goods ranging from wheel weights to cosmetics to children's products. Lead is a known human neurotoxin believed unsafe in any amount. The EPA lists a litany of health problems linked to lead, including brain and nervous system damage, behavior and learning problems, hyperactivity, slowed growth, hearing problems, reproductive problems and nerve disorders (EPA 2009a).

Mercury - is a pollutant from coal-fired power plants and other industrial sources, also used in consumer products such as fluorescent light bulbs and thermometers. It is readily converted to the organic compound methylmercury, which accumulates in the food chain, especially seafood. Eating methylmercury-tainted seafood is typically the primary source of contamination. Mercury dental fillings are a lesser source of contamination. Mercury is a neurotoxin that interferes with brain and nervous system development and is particularly harmful to the fetus, infants and children.

Dioxins and furans (chlorinated and brominated) - Dioxins and furans are contaminants in brominated flame retardants used in foam, pads, furniture, and other products. They enter the body from contaminated air, food and water. Dioxans and furans are known human carcinogens. Animal studies suggest other health risks, including endocrine disruption and immune suppression.

Polybrominated diphenyl ether (PBDEs) brominated fire retardants found in electronics, fabric, foam, furniture and plastics. They gradually migrate out of consumer products, contaminating house dust. Meat, poultry, dairy products and fish are sometimes contaminated by processing and packaging. PBDEs are considered developmental neurotoxins and can interfere with formation of thyroid hormones critical to fetal and infant brain development, and may affect children's cognitive abilities and behavior. They may also contribute to thyroid disease in adults.

PCBs (polychlorinated biphenyl ethers) - There are more than 200 PCB chemicals. Some are thin, light-colored liquids, others are yellow or black waxy solids. PCBs have been used in many industrial applications, including as transformer insulators and fire retardants, and in pesticides, paints, plastics and caulk. PCBs enter the food chain in various ways, including migration from packaging, contamination of animal feed and accumulation in fatty tissues of animals. PCBs have been classified as

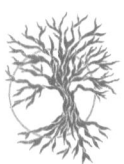

probable carcinogens and are known to be toxic to the immune, nervous and endocrine systems. They are associated with decreased alertness, responsiveness and other attention-associated behavioral measures in infants, including effects on self-quieting and motor control (Sagiv 2009).

Tetrabromobisphenol A (TBBPA), brominated fire retardant - found in electronics, carpet padding and plastic casings for televisions and computers. TBBPA is released from electronics and plastics over time. Consumption of contaminated food and, to a lesser extent, house dust contribute to human exposure. TBBPA can disrupt thyroid hormone balance.

Tonalide and Galaxolide Musk Fragrances - synthetic fragrances which are members of a large family of natural and synthetic compounds. – The Industry uses 9,000 tons of synthetic musks annually worldwide. People absorb musks through the skin, from soap, cosmetics and clothes washed with scented detergent, and by inhalation from perfumes and cologne sprays. Musks contaminate rivers, pollute fish, concentrate in body fat and persist in tissues long after exposure. A few lab studies, suggest Tonalide and Galaxolide disrupt hormones and damage organisms' defenses, allowing more toxins to seep into body cells.

Polychlorinated naphthalenes (PCNs) are found in wood preservatives, varnishes and industrial lubricants. Occupational exposure to PCNs has been associated with liver cirrhosis. Animal studies suggest that PCNs may disrupt hormone systems.

It is important to know that Chemical Mixtures Biomonitoring research such as EWG's minority cord blood study show that real world exposures do not occur chemical by chemical. Rather, each of us encounters complex mixtures of chemicals. Many of these compounds are associated with a myriad of toxicities. There are little or no data on how chemical mixtures may affect human health.

Appendix B

12 Key Additives to Avoid and Their Health Risks, (Haas, 1996)

Hydrogenated Fats—cardiovascular disease, obesity
Artificial Food Colors; allergies, asthma, hyperactivity; possible carcinogen.
Nitrites and Nitrates—these substances can develop into nitrosamines in body, which can be carcinogenic.

Sulfites (sulfur dioxide, metabisulfites, and others)—allergic and asthmatic reactions

Sugar & Sweeteners—obesity, dental cavities, diabetes and hypoglycemia, increased triglycerides (blood fats) or candida (yeast)

Artificial Sweeteners (Aspartame, Acesulfame K and Saccharin)—behavioral problems, hyperactivity, allergies, and possibly carcinogenic. The government cautions against the use of any artificial sweetener by children and pregnant women. Anyone with PKU (phenylketonuria—a problem of phenylalanine, an amino acid, metabolism) should not use aspartame (NutraSweet).

MSG (monosodium glutamate)—common allergic and behavioral reactions, including headaches, dizziness, chest pains, depression and mood swings; also, a possible neurotoxin

Preservatives (BHA, BHT, EDTA, etc.)—allergic reactions, hyperactivity, possibly cancer-causing; BHT may be toxic to the nervous system and the liver
Artificial Flavors—allergic or behavioral reactions

Refined Flour—low-nutrient calories, carbohydrate imbalances, altered insulin production

Salt (excessive)—fluid retention and blood pressure increases

Olestra (an artificial fat)—diarrhea and digestive disturbances

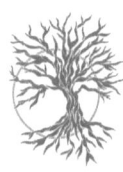

APPENDIX C
EWG CLEAN 15 and DIRTY DOZEN

The Dirty Dozen, always buy organic.

THE DIRTY DOZEN	CLEAN FIFTEEN
Strawberries	Avocadoes
Apples	Corn
Nectarines	Pineapples
Peaches	Cabbage
Celery	Sweat peas
Grapes	Onions
Cherries	Asparagus
Spinach	Mangoes
Tomatoes	Papaya
Bell peppers	Kiwi
Cherry tomatoes	Eggplant
Cucumbers	Honeydew melon
	Grapefruit
	Cantaloupe
	Cauliflower

References

Bauchuber, M. (2015) Increasing Benzodiazepine Prescriptions and Overdose Mortality in the United States 1996-2013
http://ajph.aphapublications.org/doi/full/10.2105/AJPH.2016.303061

Barrett, J. (2007). Hyperactive Ingredients. *Environmental Health Perspective*, 578.

Bearer, C. F. (1995). *Environmental* Health Hazards; how children are different from adults. *The future of Children*, 11-26.

Black, D. C. (2001). The Iowa follow-up of chemically sensitve persons. *Annals of the New York Academy of Sciences, 933* , 48-56.

Bolognesi, C., & F.D., M. (2011). Pesticides: Human Health Effects. In J. Nriagu, *Encylopedia of Environmental Health* (pp. 438-453). Genoa, Italy.

Bouchard, M. F., Bellinger, D. P., Wright, R. O., & Weisskoph, M. G. (2010). Attention-Deficit/Hyperactivity Disorder and Urinary Metabolites of Organophospate Pesticides. *Pediatrics Vol 125 ,No 6, June,* , 1270-1277.

Bridges, B. (2002). Fragrance: emerging health and *Environmental* concerns. *Flavour and Fragrance Journal. vol 17* , 361 - 371.

Burstyn, V., & Sampson, G. (2005). Techno- *Environmental* Assaults on Childhood in America. In S. P. Olfman, *Childhood Lost.* New York: Praeger Publishers.

Care2Healhy Living:
http://www.care2.com/greenliving/health-risks-of-eating-gmo-foods.html

Carter, R. (2015) Open Dialogue; A Care Model That Could Put Mental Health Social Work back on the Map. www.communitycare.co.uk/2015/02/12

CDC Autism Spectrum Disorder; https://www.cdc.gov/ncbddd/autism/data.html

CDC Features-Treatment works: Get Help for Depression and Anxiety. (2008, December 22). Retrieved July 30, 2011, from Center for Disease Control: http://www.cdc.gov/features/depression

CDC "Prescription Painkiller Overdoses at Epidemic Levels,"
http://www.cdc.gov/media/releases/2011/p1101_flu_pain_killer_overdose.html

Colbert, J. M. (2001). *Toxic Relief; Restore health and energy through fasting and detoxification.* Lake Mary: Siloam.

Deirdre Imus, (2011) Remembering Childhood Cancer Month
http://www.foxnews.com/health/2011/09/12/remembering-national-childhood-cancer-month.html#ixzz1Xn6Ueo7T

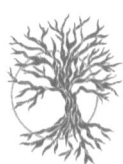

EPA. (2002, January). *Pesticides; Topical and Chemical Fact Sheets.* Retrieved from EPA: http://www.epa.gov/opp00001/factsheets/kidpesticide.htm

Frack, L., Sutton, B., (2010) *3163 Ingredients Hide behind the word Fragrance.* http://www.ewg.org/enviroblog/2010/02/3163-ingredients-hide-behind-word-fragrance

Genuis, S. J. (2008). Medical Practice and community health care in the 21st Century: A time of change. *Public Health.*

Group, E. W. (2009). *Pollution in People - Cord Blood Contaminents in Minority Newborns.*

Haas, E. D. (1996). *Staying Healthy Shoppers Guide: Feed your family safely.*

Heller, S. P. (2010). *Anxiety; Hidden Causes, why your anxiety may not be all in your head but from something physical.* Del Ray Beach: Symmetry.

Koger, S. M., Schettler, T., & Weiss, B. (2005). Environmental Toxicants and Developmental Disabilities: A Challange for Psychologists. *American Psycologist, Vol 60(3) April, ,* 243-255.

LIVING NON GMO: http://livingnongmo.org/learn/gmo-faq/

Lu, C., Toepel, K., Irish, R. F., Barr, D., & Bravo, R. (2006). Organic Diets Significantly Lower Children's Dietary Exposure to Organophosphorus Pesticides. *Enviornmental Health Perspectives, February ,* 260-263.

Lundberg, A. (1998). Introduction. In A. Lundberg, *The Environment and Mental Health* (pp. 1-4). New York: Routledge.

Martin, K. (2017) Monsanto's Glyphosate Fatty Disease Link Proven -Published-Peer Reviewed, Scrutinized Study. http://www.organiclifestylemagazine.com/monsantos-glyphosate-fatty-liver-disease-link-proven-published-peer-reviewed-scrutinized-study.

Mercola, Hidden Dangers of Aspertame. http://www.mercola.com/article/aspartame/hidden_dangers.htm

Miller C.S., M. H. (1995). Chemical Sensitivity attributed to pesticide exposure versus remodeling. *Archives of Enviornmental Health; 50 ,* 119-120.

Miller, C. M. (September 2008). The New Tapestry of Risk Assessment. *Neurotoxicology ,* 883-890.

Miller, C. (2001). The Compelling Anomaly of Chemical Intolerance. *Annals of the New York Academy of Sciences* , 1-23.

Morrison, J. A. (2011). *Cleanse your body clear your mind; eliminate environmental toxins to loose weight, increase engergy and reverse illness.* New York: Hudson Street Press.

NHMH-NIMH Statistics. Retrieved January 2017, from National Institute of Mental Health: https://www.nimh.nih.gov/health/statistics/index.shtml

Niemark, J (2013). Extreme Chemical Sensitivity Makes Suffers allergic to life. *Discover Magazine, November 2013.*

Nimmermark, S. (2004). Odour Influence on Well-Being and Health with specific focus on animal production emissions. *Agricultural Environmental Medicine (II), Swedish Unversity of Agricultural Sciences.* , 163-173.

Owens, K., Feldman, J., & Kepner., P. Wide Range of Diseases Linked to Pesticides. *Pesticides and You Vol 30, No 2, Summer 2010.*

Palmer, R. F., Blanchad, S., Stein, Z., Mandell, D., & Miller, C. (2006). Environmental mercury release, special education rates and autism disorder: an ecological study of Texas. *Health & Place Volume 12, Issue 2 June,* 203-209.

Physicians, Social Responsibility (2000). *In Harms Way: Toxic Threats to Child Development.* Boston: Greater Boston's Physicians for Social Responsiblity.

Potera, C. (2010). The Artificial Food Dye Blues. *Environmental Health Perspective* , 118.

Potera, C. (2005). The Sweet Scent on Baby's Breath. *Environmental Health Perspective* , 115.

Ranheim, P. M. (2008). *American Academy of Environmental Medicine Reaction to Nighline Program of March 20, 2008.* Retrieved July 28, 2011, from American Academy of Environmental Medicine: http://www.aaemonline.org/images/abcresponse.pd

Release, E. N. (2011). *Prenatal Pesticide Exposure Linked to Diminished IQ.* Washington DC: Environmental Working Group.

Schettler, T., & Stein, F. R. (2000). *In Harm's Way; Toxic threats to child Devleopment.* Boston: Greater Boston Physicians for Social Responsibility.

Schroeder, S. (2000). Mental retardation and developmental disabilites influenced by environmental neurotoxic insults. *Environmental Health Perspective, June 108(suppl3)* , 395-399.

Shukla, Mukta M, Ashok K; posted Jan 10, 2012. http://www.americanlaboratory.com/914-Application-Notes/37318-A-Look-Into-the-Petrochemicals-Industry/

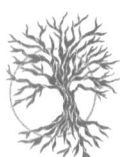

Steineman, A. C. (2016). Fragranced consumer products; exposures and effects from emissions . *Air Qual Atmos Health published OnLine October 2016*

Steineman, A. C. (2010). Fragranced consumer products; chemicals emitted, ingrediants unlisted. *Environmental Impact assessment review, August* .

Steinemann, A. C. (2008). Fragranced Consumer Products and undisclosed ingredients. *Environmental Impact Assessment Review* .

Suzuki Foundation (2017). http://www.davidsuzuki.org/issues/health/science/toxics/fragrance-and-parfum

Suzuki Foundation – Queen of Green. http://www.davidsuzuki.org/publications/resources/2011/green-cleaning-recipes/

Tilson, H., & Cabe, P. (1978). Strategy for the assessment of neurobehavioral consequenses of *environmental* factors. *Environmental Health Perspectives* , 287-299.

Toxic Chilren How US Babies became born Pre-polluted. (n.d.). Retrieved February 14, 2010, from Autism One: http://www.autismone.org/content/toxic-children-how-us-babies-became-born-pre-polluted-and-what-can-be-done-fix-silent-insidi

Walton, Ralph G. (1993). Adverse Reactions to Aspartame; Double Blind Challenge in Patients From a Vulnerable Population," Biological Psychiatry, Vol 34, pp 13 – 17.

Watch, N. E. (2004). *First Round of Results from a Study on Toxic Body Burdens.* Seattle: Northwestern *Environmental* Watch.

Weiss, B. (1998). Behavioral Manifestations of Neurotoxicity. In Lundeberg, *Ante* (pp. 25-41). New York: Routledge.

Weiss, B. (2000). Vulnerability of children and the developing brain to neurotoxic hazards. *Environmental Health Perspective; 108* , 378-381.

Whelan, L. (2015). Sales of ADHD Meds are Skyrocketing; Here's Why" Mother Jones. Http:www.motherjones.com/environment/2015/02/Hyperactive-Growth-ADHD-Medication-sales.

Wright, R. J. (2009). Moving towards making social toxins mainstream in childrens enviornmental health. *Current Opinion Pedatric* , 222-229.

Zimmerman, K. (2016) Endocrine System: Facts, Functions and Diseases. *Live   Science, March 11, 2016*

www.ingramcontent.com/pod-product-compliance
Lightning Source LLC
Chambersburg PA
CBHW050455290526
45786CB00006B/2296